mid
life

Look Younger, Live Longer & Feel Better

mid life

Look Younger, Live Longer & Feel Better

DR. MUIR GRAY

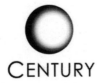

CENTURY

1 3 5 7 9 10 8 6 4 2

Century
20 Vauxhall Bridge Road
London SW1V 2SA

Century is part of the Penguin Random House group of companies
whose addresses can be found at global.penguinrandomhouse.com.

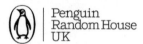

Copyright © Sir Muir Gray
Illustrations © David Mostyn

First published by Century in 2016

www.penguin.co.uk

A CIP catalogue record for this book is available from the British Library.

ISBN 9781780896625

Set in 12.25/15 pt Dante MT Std
Typeset by Jouve (UK), Milton Keynes
Printed and bound by Clays Ltd, St Ives plc

Penguin Random House is committed to a sustainable
future for our business, our readers and our planet. This book is
made from Forest Stewardship Council® certified paper.

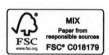

This book is dedicated to the unsung heroes of The Sandwich Generation, supporting two generations, under stress at work and giving insufficient priority to their own wellbeing.

Contents

Foreword

As Chief Medical Officer, I commonly look at health issues and risk factors that affect the entire population. In my 2013 Annual Report, for instance, I examined infectious diseases and, in particular, the threat of antimicrobial resistance. If left unchecked, this will shake the foundations of modern medicine for us all.

There is also value in focusing on specific sections of the population to take a demographic, rather than a thematic approach. This allows me to knit together strands of evidence to form a coherent picture of the health of groups within the population, and thus influence public policy in order to improve their health. Recognising that the importance of addressing their health issues, risk factors and needs is often underemphasised, I began a piece of work in 2015 to examine the data around the health of people commonly referred to as the 'Baby Boomer' generation. My forthcoming 2015 Annual Report will describe this work and give a snapshot of health for this group.

In this context, a work such as Dr Gray's is very welcome. By promoting understanding of the health issues faced by those in midlife, it should encourage people to improve their health at this stage in life and reduce their risk of disability and dementia on reaching old age. If this were achieved, it would not only increase their quality of life but also reduce the burden on their offspring when they reach midlife themselves.

I welcome Dr Gray's work and hope you enjoy reading this book.

Professor Dame Sally C Davies FRS FMedSci
Chief Medical Officer
Department of Health, London

At 20, most of us feel immortal – or at least we act that way.

At 50 – and I've just marked that birthday – the penny has begun to drop. By then, maybe you've had a health scare. Or a close friend, or brother or sister has. At the very least, perhaps you've finally succumbed to reading glasses, you've noticed your jeans getting tighter and you're a bit less agile kicking a football around the park with your kids.

So, now's the time to smell the coffee. Muir Gray – one of our country's leading doctors – sets out smart advice in this short but compelling volume. It's packed with advice on staying healthy, enjoying life and living well. The good news? Make a few impactful lifestyle changes, and the chances are we'll be the longest-living generation in human history. Lose some weight by eating less, and better. Dial back on the booze. Walk and exercise a bit more. Get your blood pressure checked, have a bowel cancer check-up when invited, 'know your numbers' on your body mass index.

Worldwide, life expectancy is rising by five hours a day. And since the 1950s, in western countries that's mostly been due to improvements in middle-aged and older people's health. Some of that is thanks to what the NHS has done for us, but much of it depends on what we choose to do for ourselves.

Our wives, husbands and partners, our children and grand-children, are all cheering us on.

Simon Stevens

CEO of NHS England, Simon is also responsible for NHS Choices and the Diabetes Prevention and the blood pressure programmes.

Introduction

I did not own or have the use of a car until I was 28. For the first 25 years of my life, neither my family nor I had the money to run one. When I was 26 and 27, I was too busy working in hospitals to need a car. In fact, I did not even think about owning one during this time.

However, at the age of 28, I got a job which required me to use one. So I bought a second hand Vauxhall Viva van into which I could load the love of my life, my bike.

From what I had learned about health and wellbeing as a result of my medical studies and the diploma in preventive medicine that I had acquired, it seemed to me that the start of a life dominated by the car and a desk job was the start of the downhill journey.

The job I had at 28 involved two things. The first was the health education of young people and the second was organising care for the elderly. As I got to know a large number of these patients, I was struck by the huge variation in ability. Some in their eighties were very disabled and dependent on others, whereas there were people the same age who were lively, driving cars, working, and performing an invaluable role in supporting their spouse or loved one. I thought to myself, 'what made the difference?'

When I discussed this with my elderly patients it became clear that, for many, the problem was caused by disease or diseases that were not preventable. So, a bit of luck is important. However, other diseases were the same ones that we were educating, or trying to educate, young people to avoid.

The second factor was loss of fitness which, for many people, could be traced to 45 years of sitting at a desk job from about the age of 20 to 65.

I could see change happening in people from the age of 20 on. By starting an office job, the effects of sitting all day might not take effect until the forties. But, there are often many other stresses in their lives: work, children and elderly parents.

For years we have assumed that everything was plain sailing for the 'grown ups' and the medical establishment has focused on the needs of children and old people. But in recent years it has become clear that midlife is a tough time. It is also clear that people in midlife can regain lost fitness and lose weight, so they can feel better, look younger and live longer. It is also clear that the changes that are needed are also changes that will reduce the risk of problems in the years to come.

Midlife is the end of the beginning, not the beginning of the end and I wrote this book, with the help of a number of experts, to help midlifers regain control.

Sir Muir Gray

Forty to Sixty: The Midlife Challenge

Last year, a friend called me in a state of dismay. He had just had his 54th birthday and he had stopped working at his job. But rather than enjoying his freedom and doing all the things he has always wanted to do, he felt trapped. He felt defined by his age, as though his life had passed him by. This shouldn't sound unfamiliar. Maybe the same thing has happened to someone you know, or maybe it happened to you when you approached midlife.

Despite what people think, there is no age at which 'midlife' starts. Broadly speaking, though, the term is used for people who are aged between 40 and 60. But, don't worry, you won't wake up on the morning of your 40th birthday and become suddenly middle-aged. It's just a broad term that is used to identify a certain demographic. Even so, there is no escaping midlife. From books to magazine articles, blogs to news reports, everyone is talking about it and everyone seems to offer something to help you during this stage of your life. Midlife was even the focus of a recent report by the National Institute for Health and Care Excellence (NICE), the key government body advising us what does and doesn't work to improve our health.

It used to be the case that when you reached your forties or fifties, you were halfway through your working life. People were very aware and very concerned about whether or not they had 'made it', or 'would make it', or, perhaps, 'would never make it'. Often the 'it' is not quite clear. To make matters worse, they may see younger people being promoted ahead of them. The pressure that can build on people to succeed before they have retired can be overwhelming. The crisis that we're so often told about is more of a social element than a medical one. Your doctor, for example, won't diagnose you with 'the midlife crisis'. The midlife crisis has its origin in the simple three-stage model of life that has dominated much of the 20th century.

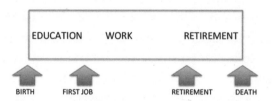

When we think about midlife or, rather, are told about midlife, it is usually partnered by the concept of 'crisis'. For many people, my friend included, midlife is the time when the heart begins to sink, the time when it looks as though it's downhill all the way to old age. But a crisis can happen at any time – it's not explicitly related to age. A career setback, an illness, a divorce or a death in the family are all events that have nothing to do with ageing. One of the popular misconceptions about midlife crises is that they are spurred by the sudden realisation that you are no longer as young as you used to be and the aspirations you once had are not achievable now you are in midlife. However, this simple three-stage model is vanishing fast as a result of dramatic changes taking place in society. The 'age of longevity' has begun. Whilst midlife is a time in which we take on new responsibilities, it is also a time to look for new adventures. Midlife is a time to be celebrated and embraced.

This book is not meant to fill you with dread, or highlight the problems with ageing. No, this book is a kick-starter. Midlife is a time to begin a new lifestyle. It is a time to make the appropriate changes in your life that will leave you feeling healthier, happier and more energetic.

People are waking up to the problems of midlife. In the past, attention has been focused on children and the elderly, and rightly so. But what about those in between? In one of her major 2016 Annual Reports, the Chief Medical Officer, Dame Sally Davies, recognised the need to highlight the midlifer which conventionally stretches from the age of about 40 to 60.

For many people, midlife is expected to be a phase of decline, with loss of fitness, weight gain and labels such as 'high blood pressure' being stuck on to add to the gloom, but this need not be the case. For people in their forties and fifties, the aim should be to get fitter, feel better, and look and feel like they did at 30. Jamie Oliver transformed his life at 40 and lost two stone; Chris Evans did it at 50, and he went to great lengths to reverse 'midlife decline' – 26 miles 385 yards to be precise, because he chose the London Marathon as a stimulus. Cameron Diaz wrote an excellent book on longevity when she became 40, and Margaret Webb wrote a powerful book on 'what women runners can teach us all about living younger, longer', telling how she and her 55-year-old sister became marathon runners. The title of her book is *Older, Faster, Stronger*.

The key is to look at midlife not as a stage of life in which you just have to try to cope better, but as a stage of development. It should be a stage in which you reflect on what you have achieved so far and then develop a plan for how you can change and adapt this for the 2020s, 2030s and 2040s.

This book is a travel guide, or a route map, to help you on that journey through your forties and fifties. After 40, you really have to look after yourself. When you're under 40, you can get away with ignoring what is happening to you (although, the ageing process actually starts in your twenties and thirties). But in the following decades you need to take action. Not against ageing, but against the three other processes that cause the problems which many people ignore because they assume that everything that happens from 40 on is due to ageing. When in reality, it's not.

Here is what many midlifers believe is happening:

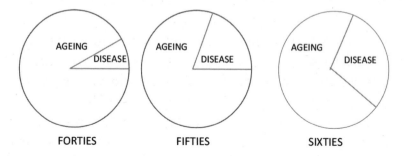

People (and this may include you) think it is all about ageing from 40 onwards, with diseases like high blood pressure creeping up and being responsible for decline. This is not the case. Ageing, as we shall see throughout this book, is relatively unimportant.

This is what happens to most people:

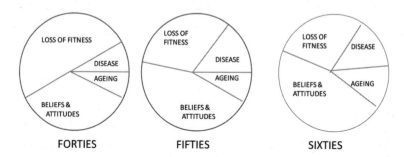

The most distinctive change is in attitude. People (and again, this might include you) go from being positive to negative and pessimistic, and this leads many people to give up looking after themselves and staying fit. Instead, midlifers give priority to other age groups – younger children or elderly parents, for example.

This book explains how to lengthen your odds, how to increase your chances of living longer and better and decrease the risk that you will come to a bad end! The bonus is that the changes you make to live longer and better will also help you feel better within weeks and you can become as fit as you were ten years ago.

The first step is to help you think about yourself. You need to reflect on where you are now and where you want to get to, not in your job but in your life. This also involves reflecting on how much pressure you are under and how you could find more time and space to look after yourself.

The second step is not to bombard you with information but to help you think about how you can reduce the stress in your life, because it is stress that makes it difficult for people to make the changes that will transform their health, now and in the future.

After that I will give you information that you can use to reduce your risk of disease and look after your body, with specific sections on:

- stress
- sleep
- exercise
- diet
- everyday health

Finally, as in any good guidebook, I will give you information about where to find help and support not only through the NHS but through many other services that can help you reduce your risk of disease and feel better.

Always remember: the most important person is you. It's time to tackle midlife.

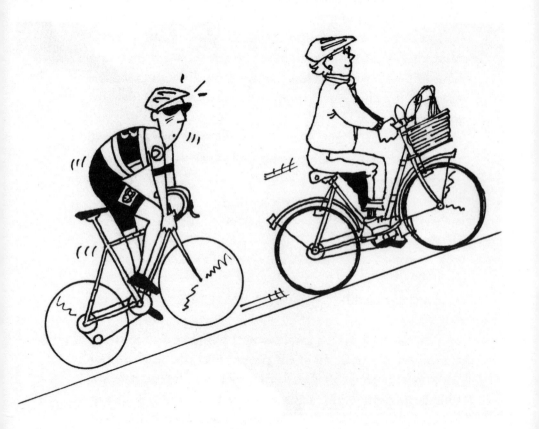

2.

The Science of Midlife

The newspapers are full of information about how people aged 40 or 50 can reduce the risk of cancer or heart disease. What newspapers fail to mention, though, is that people aged 40 or 50 (or indeed of any age) differ from one another. You are unique. The knowledge that we now have about staying healthy and reducing risk of disease has to be related to your particular circumstances. The things that you care about and the pressures that you are under are vastly different from someone else's. There is only one you and the general information about risk has to be personalised. The NHS Health Check that people over the age of 40 are offered is designed to help you relate the risks to your particular situation. It also offers testing that you cannot do yourself – a blood test, for example. In addition, the One You project launched in 2016 has an online 'How Are You?' quiz designed especially for this purpose.

This book will supplement what you will have learned, as well as help you take action, if you have had an NHS Health Check or completed the How Are You quiz. It provides you with knowledge about steps you can take which will help you stay young, feel better and live longer even if you have not had an NHS Health Check. You have to relate the information offered here to your own particular situation and turn it into useful personalised knowledge.

Firstly, here is the checklist from the online How Are You quiz. Put a ring round the number that best describes you in the range from 5 at the bottom to 1 if you feel in tip-top form.

Full of beans	1 2 3 4 5	Really knackered
Can run for miles	1 2 3 4 5	Can't run for a bus
Feeling calm	1 2 3 4 5	Totally wound up
Sleep like a baby	1 2 3 4 5	Sleepless nights
Lean and mean	1 2 3 4 5	Fat and flabby
Over the moon	1 2 3 4 5	Down in the dumps

If you scored:

- 6, that's great. Even 12 or less shows that you are doing well.
- 13 to 20, you are doing not too badly but could feel better as well as reducing the risk of long-term problems by taking action.
- 20 or more, don't despair. You can feel a great deal better and the good news is that the steps you take to reduce your risks of disease in the long term will also help you feel better within a month.

When you do the online quiz, your score starts to identify your risk profile so that it personalises the information, advice and encouragement it gives. I would suggest that you search online for 'One You' and see for yourself what you score.

For now, let's get an assessment of how you rate your health right now.

How would you rate your health now?	Put a tick here
Very good	
Good	
OK	
Bad	
Very bad	

If you rated your health as bad or very bad, what would you say is the principal cause or causes?

Possible causes of health problems	You can tick more than one box
Stress	
I have a long-term medical condition such as type 2 diabetes or asthma or high blood pressure	
I have more than one medical condition	
Poor-quality medical care	
Tiredness	
Some other reason	

Now look at the boxes that you have highlighted. If you have ticked one or more boxes, you will need to tackle the cause, or causes, directly. Think about why you feel that way and what you can do to change. Reducing your risk of disease, or getting fitter, will help you feel better overall. Even if you have one or more of the problems listed above, you can overcome them.

The proportion of people with one or more long-term conditions increases each decade. By the age of 40, roughly one-third of the population are diagnosed with one long-term condition or 'morbidity'. By 50, it is half and by 60, roughly two-thirds have at least one chronic health problem. That being said, all the information is as relevant to people with one or more long-term health problems as it is to people who do not have any.

Midlife is a tough time, but no matter how tough life is today or how pressing the problems you face, just take a few minutes to think about your future 20 or 30 years down the road.

There is a chance that you haven't thought about your future health and well-being and that's OK. Your day-to-day pleasures are important and life gets in the way. But it's important not to forget that midlife is quickly approaching. So, what do you hope or fear will happen to you in the future? Take a couple of minutes to think about this.

What are your hopes and fears for the future?	Indicate which of these you identify with most strongly
I hope to drop dead suddenly	
I hope I don't develop dementia	
I hope I won't be disabled and a burden on my family	
I hope I can stay pretty fit until pretty near the end	

Dropping dead suddenly on the last day of a wonderful holiday on which you have spent all your savings might seem to you to be a great way to go, but it has its downside. It can be very tough for those left behind, particularly if you have not told them how much you love them. Most people, however, are not obsessed with living as long as possible. It is the quality of life that is more important. Being dependent on your family for years, stuck in a chair and unable to get to the toilet in time is a miserable prospect, but the good news is that it is not inevitable. In any journey you need to decide where you are going and this is as true for the journey through life as for one behind the wheel of a car, or when buying a ticket via the Internet. Set out below are some options for your long-term destination, in particular what your last months and years may be like when they come. Put your preferences (1), (2) and (3) in the first column for what you would like to happen, and then in the second column what you think will happen.

Options	What would you like to happen to you?	What do you think will happen to you?
Stay as fit as I am now and then pop off without warning		
Stay as fit as I am now and have a good, fairly quick, death without symptoms and near to those I care about		
Be chair-bound and housebound for a couple of years, relying on others to help me wash and dress and even get to the toilet		

The first option seems the most laid-back and sensible but the probability is that if you do nothing and wait and see, you will finish up with the third option – housebound, perhaps chair-bound, and reliant on others for the tasks of daily life. We are all dependent on other people. Even the wealthiest, fittest and strongest 50-year-old is dependent on others. However, there is a difference between being dependent on telephone companies, supermarkets, airline pilots and train drivers and being 'depressingly dependent' – that is, dependent on other people for getting up, washing, bathing and getting enough to eat. But before you get depressed here are two bits of good news.

The good news is that you can change your destiny by taking action, starting now, when you are 40, 50, 60, 70 or even 80. There is also some research showing that people in their nineties can regain lost strength through training. Of course if you are under pressure and feeling the effects of stress you may be more concerned about your finances next Friday than thinking 30 years ahead. But (and here is the second piece of good news) the changes you make to help you live longer and better will not only help in the long term, they will also help you feel better in the short term.

Obviously, people who take up the offer of an NHS Health Check do so for health reasons. But that's not the only reason why people take a Health Check. Being healthy is much more than the absence of disease, so using the checklist from the How Are You quiz will help you to reflect on other reasons for trying to change.

Apart from not getting ill, what are your top 3 health priorities?	
Fitting into my jeans	
Having more energy	
Avoiding aches and pains	
Feeling young	
Staying independent	
Keeping my mind sharp	
Having a more active social life	
Staying young-looking	
Being there for my kids and grandchildren	

Fortunately what you need to do to achieve all your long-term hopes will help you feel better in the short term; not necessarily immediately but within about a month you will start feeling healthier, younger and invigorated. Many people face pressing problems in their life that make change difficult, so let's identify the principal obstacles.

The questions from the How Are You quiz help you identify some of the barriers which are stopping you overcoming your goals by asking 'What stops you taking care of yourself?' This is a useful checklist but it implies that it's your fault and that you have chosen to live in a way that is bad for your health, which isn't entirely true. As we will discover, there are some aspects which are out of your control. The modern environment has increased the risk of heart disease and type 2 diabetes. But one thing to remember is that 'ageing' or 'growing old' is not the cause of these problems.

What stops you taking care of yourself?	
I don't have the time	
It's more important I look after others	
I don't know what to do	
I don't have the money	
I start but can't keep it up	
Nothing, I take good care of myself	

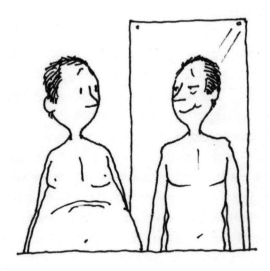

The ageing process

Sir Bradley Wiggins, at the age of 35, set a new world record for the distance cycled in an hour, 54.526 kilometres, but he probably will not set a new world record at the age of 40, no matter how hard he tries – although I hope he proves me wrong. For events which require endurance, athletes reach their peak in their early thirties if they have the right attitude, continue training and manage to escape injury. Paula Radcliffe set the women's marathon record at the age of 30, Serena Williams won Wimbledon at the age of 34 and Roger Federer, despite injury, reached the Wimbledon semi-finals for the 11th time at the same age.

Ageing is a normal biological process – to be more accurate, a set of processes – which is not fully understood. The ageing process does have an effect on many body tissues and organs which reduces your ability to do things. For example, the maximum heart rate drops by about one beat per minute every year from the age of about 35, and this is one reason why Sir Bradley is unlikely to beat his record, even if he continues to train as hard between 35 and 36 as he trained between the ages of 25 and 35.

The other consequence of the ageing process is what people term a loss of resilience, or the power of homeostasis: not just the loss of the ability to do things but the loss of the ability to bounce back and respond when something goes wrong. For example, an individual's ability to respond to losing their balance is reduced due to ageing, so a stumble may become a fall. It is inactivity that is perhaps the greatest threat that many of us face in an environment where most people spend most of the time either in bed or sitting down. Inactivity is a challenge and the effects of ageing reduce the ability to respond appropriately to inactivity.

A great deal of research is going on into ageing and there is a growing interest and investment in research to develop antidotes to ageing. The elixir of life was the name given to such an antidote by the ancients and it has played a part in fables for hundreds, perhaps thousands, of years. *The Philosopher's Stone* is part of the Harry Potter saga and the term philosopher's stone, sometimes used to describe something that could turn base metal into gold, was used on other occasions to describe the elixir of life.

There is serious money and brainpower going into this now, and that astonishing company Google has invested a lot of resources to set up a company called Calico (short for California Life Company), the aim of which is to create medicines that will keep us alive until – claims vary – the age of 142, 150, or beyond.

This type of science is leading to a new medical speciality called regenerative medicine, more advanced in the USA where the search for eternal youth has always been more ardently pursued. The Mayo Clinic website describes how their Center for Regenerative Medicine takes 'three inter-related approaches':

- **Rejuvenation.** Rejuvenation means boosting the body's natural ability to heal itself. Though after a cut your skin heals within a few days, other organs don't repair themselves as readily. But cells in the body once thought to be no longer able to divide (terminally differentiated) – including the highly specialised cells constituting the heart, lungs and nerves – have been shown to be able to remodel and possess some ability to self-heal. Teams within the center are studying how to enhance self-healing processes.
- **Replacement.** Replacement involves using healthy cells, tissues or organs from a living or deceased donor to replace damaged ones. Organ transplants, such as heart and liver transplants, are good examples.
- **Regeneration.** Regeneration involves delivering specific types of cells or cell products to diseased tissues or organs, where they will ultimately restore tissue and organ function.

In Oxford in 2016 these techniques were successfully used to treat one cause of blindness, but the journey is at an early stage so don't give up on fitness in the hope that regenerative medicine will be waiting for you. At present there is nothing I can recommend that will slow the ageing process; however, you can influence the other three processes, preventable disease, loss of fitness and a negative pessimistic attitude towards the social process of growing older, and the first step is to become more positive.

Developing the right attitude is one of the key characteristics you need to have to enjoy yourself and stay healthy. Attitude is even more important than being well informed, although that is important too. Research has shown that many people have a fatalistic attitude to what will happen to them, or have so many other problems on their plate than worrying about their diet, their level of fitness or even about why they are so stressed, that they cannot summon up the energy to try to be less stressed! Many people are facing such short-term deadlines – rent to be found for next Friday, loans to be repaid next payday, uncertainty about how many hours will be offered and therefore what the pay will be next payday – that looking after themselves is a low priority. But we know human beings are able to change, no matter how difficult the environment, and one aspect of life that needs to be encouraged is a positive attitude.

Keeping a positive attitude involves not only thinking positively inside yourself, it also means resisting and rejecting the negative attitudes of people around you.

You can close the fitness gap

Let's take the life course of someone who has had a healthy childhood, keeps as fit as possible, prevents the preventable diseases and is also lucky enough to avoid those diseases that are not preventable. Their life course is shown in the graph below. They are affected only by ageing, peak in their early thirties and then lose ability.

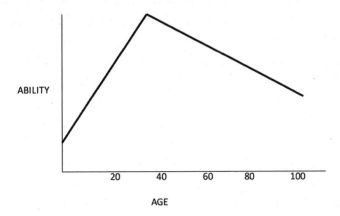

Most people, however, do not continue to develop till they peak in their thirties; only professional athletes can do that (because they are paid large sums of money to train every day). For most people, the turning point comes in their early twenties, not because of ageing but because they get their first job, become too busy to continue with sport, and start a lifetime of sitting and focusing on the here and now. Many people prefer not to think about the future at all. They adopt

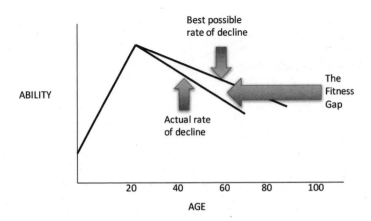

a fatalistic approach to life – what will be, will be – and hope that they will pop off quickly with a nice little heart attack. Even by keeping as fit as possible, and by following the best possible rate of decline (as shown in the graph on page 23), they will lose ability. However, what is much more likely to happen is progressive loss of fitness from the age of 20, complicated later by development of disabling diseases, because they have not bothered to take any of the opportunities to reduce their risk. A huge gap opens up between how able they are and how able they would have been had they kept fit. This is called the fitness gap.

The good news is that by taking action at the age of 40 or 50 or older, a person can change course from point A to point B as they do so, become as able and fit as they were five or ten years previously, and live much better for longer.

Another way of thinking about what has happened is that the 50-year-old person has not only closed the fitness gap, but has regained the level of fitness and ability they had when they were 40 – they have got younger!

So although you cannot slow the ageing process you can close the fitness gap, stay as young as you are, and get younger. This applies even if you develop some disease, but remember that many diseases can be prevented or postponed.

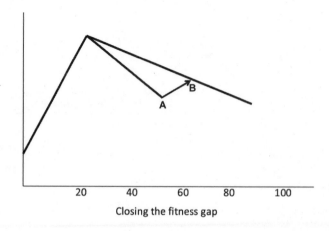

Closing the fitness gap

Preventing disease

Unlike ageing, disease is not a normal biological process. Many diseases, including dementia, can be prevented or postponed by actions taken in midlife and the steps you can take to reduce your risks are summarised in this book.

Some diseases are at present not preventable and may be due to genetic factors, but it is currently estimated that genetics are responsible for no more than one-fifth of common diseases; the other four-fifths are preventable in both men and women.

The good news is that the steps you can take to reduce your risk of disease will also help you feel better within a few weeks, so risk reduction is not just an activity that might pay off in 30 years. The same actions that reduce risk improve vitality and well-being. It is also essential to remember that one-third of people in their forties and 50 per cent of people in their fifties have already had at least one long-term condition such as type 2 diabetes or high blood pressure diagnosed and they need to try to become fitter and eat better, at least as much as people without any disease or condition.

Don't worry about your genes

Genetics is in the news every week, and there is no doubt that your genes are important. They determine the colour of your eyes, the colour of your hair, and, if you are a man, how long you will keep it. The importance of your unique genetic inheritance in deciding whether or not you develop disease is also often in the news, but how important are your genes?

In general, it seems that genes are less important than the environment in which you grow up and live, and the way you adapt to it. The expectation of life of people in the United

Kingdom increased by eight years between 1990 and 2010, and there is no way in which this could have been brought about by genetic evolution. Similarly, there is still an eight-year difference in life expectancy between people who live in the wealthiest part of the country and those who live in the poorest part of the country, and there is no way this can be explained by genetic evolution. The international differences in health between different countries are more the result of differences in lifestyle and environment than the result of genetic differences.

But what about you, an individual with your unique genetic code? Firstly, you need to understand that there are two ways in which genes affect your risk of disease. You have millions of genes but the risk of some diseases are determined by the presence or absence of a single gene. Most publicity has been given to the BRCA genes, BRCA 1 and BRCA 2, which dramatically increase the risk of breast cancer. There are, however, two other common diseases in which the risk is greatly increased by a single gene – bowel cancer and heart disease.

There are two ways in which the risk of these diseases can be detected. Firstly, the NHS tries to contact the relatives of people diagnosed with

- Breast cancer and the BRCA gene
- Bowel cancer as a result of a genetic disorder called the Lynch Syndrome
- Familial hypercholesterolaemia – very, very high levels of cholesterol because of a genetic deficiency

NHS Choices also has very clear information on these genes and conditions.

The other approach is what you can do for yourself. Obviously you cannot change your genetic inheritance at present as changing your genetic code is science fiction. But you can be aware of the possibility that you might be at high risk and ask for a genetic test if you have one or more close family members who have developed one of the following diseases before the age of 50:

- Bowel cancer (cancer of the colon)
- Breast cancer
- Prostate cancer
- A heart attack

Ask your GP for a blood test and referral to a specialist centre.

There are also a large number of rare diseases, which are too large to mention individually, that are passed on genetically by a single gene disorder. However, services for these rare conditions are often well organised, partly because the people who suffer from them have set up charities to provide help and support for sufferers. These conditions are defined as 'rare' which means that a GP may never encounter someone with the condition in their whole career, and even a specialist in a hospital might see very few patients because all the people with the condition are referred to a few super-specialist services.

So much for the diseases caused by a single gene. The genetic information is relatively straightforward to understand and act on. What is developing, however, is a mass of information about common conditions such as type 2 diabetes, stroke, Alzheimer's disease, and arthritis. Initially, there was terrific excitement in the scientific community because of the prospect of finding the gene defect that led to arthritis. However, what is emerging as more research is carried out, is that there are no single genes for these common problems. There are tens or hundreds, or perhaps thousands, of genes that play a part in determining your level of risk. So genetic tests for those conditions do not appear to add much value to the simpler biochemical tests that have been used for years, for example testing blood sugar to assess the risk of type 2 diabetes.

There is no doubt that genetic advances will help the battle against common diseases, and they are already doing so. We should therefore support genetic research, which is making big advances in understanding how bacteria evolve and how the cunning little devils evolve resistance to antibiotics so quickly and effectively. It is certainly essential that we use less antibiotics in medicine and, even more important, in agriculture, but it is also essential to pursue the genetic line of attack on bacteria. Secondly, genetic research is helping us understand how to choose the drug that is right for you, namely the drug that has the highest chance of doing good and the lowest chance of doing harm.

Up to now we have talked about high blood pressure or type 2 diabetes, or breast cancer as though they were single conditions. In fact, it is more accurate to talk about breast cancers because there are many types of breast cancer. They look the same on the x-ray or to the surgeon's eye, but the genetic make-up of the cancer – the way in which the genetic pattern of the normal cancer cell has gone mad and multiplied without control, is not always the same. In the past, we had to offer all women with breast cancer the same drug even though we knew that a proportion of them would not get any benefit but that they would be at equal risk of side-effects as the women who did benefit. Now there is a genetic test that can identify which women have the type of cancer that will not respond to this particular drug, so many women will be spared the side-effects from a drug that is ineffective for them.

This is all part of a trend called 'personalisation' in the move from what has been called production line medicine, when all patients get the same treatment. Obviously the tests and treatments that people are offered should all be of the same high quality and effectiveness. However, every individual is unique, both genetically and psychologically, and these high-quality components need to be put together in a way that recognises this. Just as every car can be configured to meet the specification of the person who has ordered it, so every medical treatment needs to be designed and delivered to meet your needs.

Firstly, of course, you need to be clear about what you want from life and health, and that is the aim of this book.

Develop your assets

If you are a millionaire, your assets are obvious – your yacht, your private jet, your penthouse suite. But even those who are not millionaires will still have some assets – maybe you have a house, a car or cash in the bank. These are your tangible assets: the things you can see and sometimes touch. You will also have intangible assets, however. These are things that you cannot touch but that are equally important. It is these assets which this book will focus on. I will show you how you can improve your health and vitality. Throughout the book, I will also be telling you to focus on two types of intangible assets: productive and transformational. These assets are described in a book by Lynda Gratton and Andrew Scott called *The 100 Year Life* in which they emphasise that the traditional life with retirement at 65 (earlier if you were lucky) is vanishing. It is being replaced by a world in which many people will live till they are 100, and work until they are 80. In midlife people would reinvent themselves and build on and develop their intangible assets.

Your productive assets are your knowledge and skills. You will need to think about the skills that have stood you well and think about the changes that are taking place at your workplace. As they say in the army when things have gone awry, you need to regroup. Perhaps you need to acquire new skills? Or perhaps you need to gather more knowledge? Whatever it is you need to do to succeed, you will be able to learn a new set of concepts and skills. Middle-aged people make great students and often organise their time and studies better. Someone once said: 'University is wasted on the young.'

'"Transformational assets" refers to your self-knowledge, the ability to reach out into diverse networks and openness to new experiences.' These can be improved in various ways. Volunteering is one of them. By volunteering with challenging groups of people (in a prison, for example), or running for political office in your local council, you will be open to new ideas and new experiences. By reaching out to the community, you can even reduce stress, learn new skills and advance your career. In 2016 midlife internships were launched. Primarily for women returning from five or ten years of parenting, they are relevant to anyone considering a significant change in their journey. Perhaps you're interested in moving to a different occupation from that which you have occupied for 20 years of your working life, or maybe you just want to experience something new. Internships are no longer something for university graduates. So, instead of thinking about recreation, which implies hobbies and activities which help you relax, think about re-creation.

Midlife is not the beginning of the end, but the end of the beginning.

Part One

Reducing Stress

Resources on reducing stress	What's in it for you
Health Check	Stress is not covered in the Health Check but you can ask the nurse about stress if you feel this is a factor affecting your behaviour
One You	The How Are You quiz asks you to identify any pressures that might make it difficult for you to look after your health, for example by asking if you don't have enough money or enough time
Your annual review if you have a long-term condition like type 2 diabetes or high blood pressure	The person carrying out the review should ask how you are feeling about the condition that is being reviewed. They should be interested in how much stress is being caused by your condition and how much stress from that, or any other cause, interferes with your coping with the condition
NHS Choices	NHS Choices has checklists to help you assess your level of stress and techniques that you can use to reduce it
High-quality apps	Try the Stress Check app

When you are a parent of young children, it is clear what your mission is. People understand and sympathise with the pressures that you're under and what is causing stress and anxiety. However, the stresses and pressures of midlife are much less clear. They can be emotional or physical, or both.

Generally, the word 'stress' is used broadly for when things get too much – when you are overloaded with pressure and you can't cope. That pressure can come from numerous outlets – family, financial difficulties, work-related problems. The list is endless and will, eventually, lead to stress.

But what is stress and what can you do to prevent it? Statements like 'I'm stressed' or 'I have a high-stress job' might sound familiar and you may have said them yourself. This makes stress sound as though it's something external. When actually, stress is something within you.

NHS Choices defines stress as 'the feeling of being under too much mental or emotional pressure. Pressure turns into stress when you feel unable to cope. People have different ways of reacting to stress, so a situation that feels stressful to one person may be motivating to someone else.'

So stress is internal, but it is a reaction to external factors. An unreasonable and demanding boss, financial problems that require a difficult decision, disagreement with your

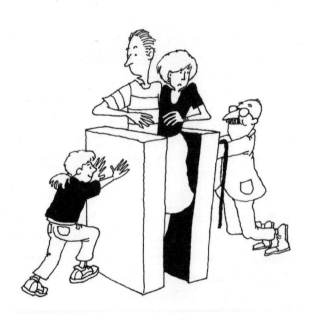

partner or with teenage children, or problems with your parents – these are all external factors that can lead to stress. The feeling we get is not only psychological, but also physical.

Doctors have been reluctant to help patients tackle stress or even discuss it because the scientific study of stress has not produced research findings as clear-cut as research on smoking. But it is clear now that stress increases your risk of a bad end both directly and because stress from work or family life makes it difficult to get fitter or eat better. Of course, suddenly being told that you have a condition like high blood pressure itself causes stress, so let's think how you can cope with and reduce stress as the first step on the road to better health for longer.

The problem now is that the stressors in our life are not the type of danger that requires physical activity; rather, they generate a mental or emotional reaction. A modern definition of stress is, therefore, a feeling of being under too much social or emotional pressure. Part of the problem is that there is no simple solution. Modern stress is chronic, long term and harmful, with effects on your mind and body that make you feel bad and increase the risk of, or aggravate, a number of important health problems all caused by chronic inflammation.

However, compared to women, men appear to find discussing these issues with each other more difficult. Matthew Solan, the executive editor of the *Harvard Men's Health Watch*, writes in 'A Guide to Men's Health 50 and Forward':

Speaking for my gender, there are two qualities that define most men: we seldom like to ask for help, and we do not like to talk about our feelings. Combining the two – asking for help about our feelings – is the ultimate affront to many men's masculinity.

Conversations between men are different from conversations between women. For men, the midlife crisis often focuses on work-related anxieties. Later in this section, I will emphasise the importance of recognising that midlife is a stage of transition and the result can be depression.

Feeling stress is not a sign of weakness, but some people are afraid to speak about their feelings for fear that their boss or colleagues, who may be feeling just the same, will talk about them 'not coping'. You can diagnose the stress reaction by being aware of one or more of the symptoms below:

- A feeling of mild panic, for example that you will never get through the day's work or even the day's emails
- Muscular tension in your jaw
- Sweating, even when the outside temperature is not very hot
- Grumbling guts with some mixture of upper abdominal pain, diarrhoea and constipation
- Difficulty in sleeping

Now, using the table below, record how often you feel one or more of the symptoms listed above.

How often do you feel these symptoms of stress?	Tick if this applies to you
Never	
About once a month	
Once a week	
More days than not	
Every day	

You are a lucky person if you have ticked the 'Never' box because very few people in their forties and fifties lead the type of life in which there is no emotional or psychological pressure. Even if you do not feel the symptoms of stress in the list above, there are behaviours that the *Harvard Medical School Special Health Report on Stress Management* recognises and if you behave in two of the ways listed below you should think about stress being a problem for you.

- Are you frequently late?
- Are you often angry or irritated?
- Are you showing inability to do something?
- Do you feel overextended?
- Do you tell us that you 'don't have enough time for stress relief'?
- Do you feel a little bit tense?
- Do you often feel pessimistic?
- Are you upset by conflict with others?
- Do you feel worn out or burnt out?
- Do you feel lonely?

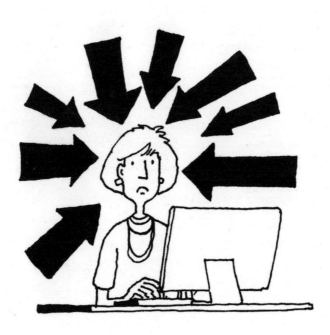

The mind and brain are like software and hardware. The mind is the software – a complicated operating system full of little programs. You might have installed some of these programs yourself, but others (like viruses or malware) have been installed by other people.

The mind operates at a great rate in childhood, but there is no age at which the mind cannot change or develop further. But, and this is important, *you* need to decide to develop it. In midlife, your mind will change whether you try to influence that process or not, so it is much better to take charge than let it happen at the direction of other people.

Obviously the hardware, your brain, is important too and you need to take some steps to make sure your brain stays as healthy as possible, and everything we know about the brain is similar to our bodily organs: ageing isn't important. Professor Carol Brayne in Cambridge has discovered that dementia, something previously thought to be a complication of ageing, is now considered to be a result of lifestyle and environmental problems that lead to stress and loss of fitness.

The first step, as always, is to try to reduce the external pressures that stimulate the stress reaction. What are the pressures that make it difficult for you to look out for yourself a little better?

Common pressures	Indicate which put pressure on you
Problems with children	
Problems with parents	
Uncertainty about where you are going in your life	
Relationship problems	
Housing problems, cost or insecurity	
Financial problems	
Pressures at work	

Some of these are very difficult to tackle. Low income may be completely out of your control, as may be housing difficulties, but some of these pressures are within your power to influence. For example, midlife is a time when separation and divorce become more common and there are few generators of stress more powerful than divorce and the tension leading up to it. However, divorce is not inevitable when relationships start to change. It is often possible to resolve difficulties when you and your partner communicate more and discuss the problems surrounding your relationship. Midlife is a time to take stock – to think about where you are and where you want to be. As we've already seen, midlife is a time of transition in which you need to reflect on everything. This might be happening either to you alone, or to both of you. What's important is that when problems start to develop, you look for advice and support. It should be acknowledged that you are different people from the people who were married or paired up in your mid-twenties.

Stress is not a sign of personal weakness. It is caused by the environment in which we live and there are two aspects of modern life that are particularly harmful: one is the pressure under which many people live, the other is the fact that we often have to face stress when we are immobile, sitting at a desk in an office facing an unfair manager or at a counter dealing with an angry customer.

If you cannot solve the problems that are causing the stress reaction, there are techniques to reduce the impact these problems – the stressors – have on the stress reaction inside you, and there is now a new strategy to help people cope with stress.

It used to be that people's response to stress was either to do nothing or to visit their GP. The former course of action is not recommended and simply leads to further trouble, as stress is a vicious cycle. The second course of action, going to the GP, might be helpful but in the average consultation – about 12 minutes – there is little the GP can do to get to the root of the problem. The outcome of such visits was the prescription of a drug for depression or anxiety and words of encouragement to try to relax more.

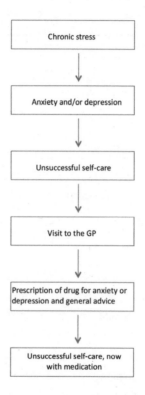

There is now agreement in the medical field that this approach is unlikely to be successful and a different system is needed, which starts by helping the person affected to cope successfully.

GPs now have other things they can do to help you to combat stress. They can give advice on how to relax using techniques developed by clinical psychologists and they can also refer you to a psychology service. This is not the same as being referred to a psychiatrist and does not indicate that you are mentally ill. Psychologists are trained to teach people how to cope with stress and its consequences, not with drugs, but by thinking differently and using techniques that we will examine briefly below and which are described in more detail on the NHS Choices website. You can try these yourself before going to the GP.

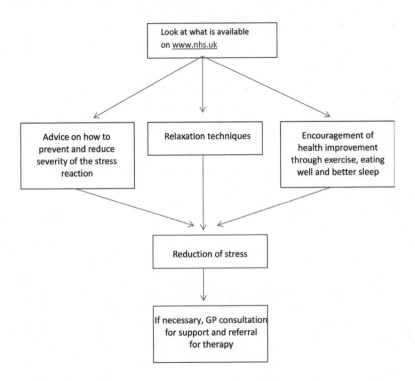

The effect of problems at work and in the family can be lessened by adopting some simple techniques based on the research of people like Professor Cary Cooper. Cooper, the key adviser to NHS Choices, has made the study of stress, its prevention and mitigation, his life's work.

These techniques will reduce the external pressures and problems that trigger the stress reaction and keep it going. However, no matter how well organised you are, you may develop stress and there is growing interest in steps you can take yourself, other than more caffeine or more alcohol, to relax and switch off the stress reaction.

Technique	How to
Do not use generalisations such as 'you always find fault with me and me alone'	Think before you speak and be careful before you use the word 'always' or 'never'
Set clear achievable goals	Make a list of jobs for the day and the week
Organise your time better	Make a timetable of the jobs that have to be done, giving each an allotted period of time
Work smarter, not longer	When you have a stressful task coming up, dealing with a difficult boss or colleague, for example, plan and rehearse beforehand

The effects of the stress reaction are to make you ready for whatever might occur and that means increasing alertness and the tension in your muscles. It would not be very helpful if, in times of danger, you became sleepier and more relaxed. So you need to learn how to relax, not by going to the pub or taking a holiday, but to relax in two minutes at work when you are in your department or when standing in a bus queue, or even standing in a bus because there are no seats. Harvard Medical School and NHS Choices recommend a number of techniques to help you relax. The Harvard recommendations are based on their research at the world-famous Institute for Mind and Body Medicine. You can learn how to do these for even a short period of time although in general the longer the better.

Technique	How to do it – more information and examples on www.nhs.uk	Time needed
Relaxed breathing	Breathe in and out slowly and deeply, saying 'breathe in, breathe out' to yourself as you do so. You need to learn how to do what is called diaphragmatic breathing. Instead of sucking your stomach in and puffing your chest out, try to let your abdominal muscles relax and bulge forward as you breathe in; this allows the diaphragm, the muscle between the chest and the abdomen, to fall and expand every bit of your lungs	1 minute
Deep muscle relaxation	In a chair, consciously relax the muscles of first your lower limbs, then your arms, chest and shoulders and finally your neck, turning it gently from side to side. Don't slump – keep your posture good but relax	3 minutes
Mindfulness	See the NHS Choices page on mindfulness, which helps you learn how to switch off from the immediate pressures of work or home and take five minutes to get a stable, calm view of the world	5 minutes
Prayer	For believers, prayer is very helpful	1 minute

(continued)

Technique	How to do it – more information and examples on www.nhs.uk	Time needed
Yoga, tai chi, Pilates or Alexander technique	Attending a class is good to learn techniques that you can use yourself between the classes. There are also examples of exercises for all these techniques you can safely try on NHS Choices and I say more about them in my section on health services that you can access directly	3 minutes

These are all good techniques to employ if you become tense as a result of the stress reaction. If you want to learn two simple techniques, NHS Choices has a web page with clear advice on relaxed breathing and deep muscle relaxation, as well as its pages on mindfulness, yoga, tai chi and Pilates.

Both the relaxation and the preventive techniques are more effective if you are generally in fairly good shape. All of these techniques – preventive, relaxing and adaptive – require time, of course, and you need to work out ways to create even small windows for what Professor Cooper calls 'me time'. It is now recognised that many people are caught in a vicious cycle in which they feel unfit, tired, unhealthy and stressed, and maybe assume that everything is due to 'getting older'. But it's not. The aim of the One You and the Health Check programmes is to help you identify how you could make changes for better health, but both recognise that for many people the main obstacle they face is stress within them.

You need a two-pronged attack, one on stress and the other on those factors that make you feel less than 100 per cent now and increase your risk of early disability and death.

These steps are just as relevant to you if you already have a long-term condition like bronchitis or high blood pressure. Just as you need to take care of your body to prevent and manage physical problems, you need to take care of your mind to prevent or deal with the big two common problems – anxiety and depression.

Anxiety and depression often coincide with one another, whilst stress can lead to anxiety or depression. It is important to remember that each condition can overlap with another, or could appear on its own.

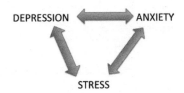

Depression is an important issue (not least because the risk of suicide is greatly increased). Some people have had depression for years or decades, but for others, depression occurs for the first time in midlife. Earlier, we talked about the 'midlife crisis', and depression can be an effect of this.

Depression is common. Indeed, if you met someone aged between 40 and 60 who said that they had never been depressed or suffered from depression, you would wonder. One way to think about depression is to ask if there is an obvious cause, because it is reasonable to be depressed in the middle of a messy divorce, or after having been made redundant, or when you have money problems, or for a million other reasons. If you start feeling depressed, or someone you know is depressed, then you need the support of friends and family.

Depression is now being taken much more seriously in the medical field. If you or someone you know is suffering from depression, then here are some simple guidelines: depression is a particularly important problem because of the risk of suicide and the risk in men is now being taken much more seriously because of the difficulty that men have in expressing what they feel or seeking help. The brilliant book *Manage your Mind* by Gillian Butler and Tony Hope is based on two basic principles – value yourself more highly and recognise that you can change.

There are also seven basic skills described in the book:

- Manage yourself and your time better
- Face up to problems and take action at an early stage
- Treat yourself well
- Be active in problem solving
- Keep things in perspective
- Continue to build your self-confidence and self-esteem
- Learn how to relax

The book contains 470 pages of distilled wisdom based on two lifetimes of clinical work and research by the authors. It covers a wide range of techniques designed to prevent, solve or reduce the problems you face. The basic message is that problems in the mind which may be primarily about how you think about things or about how you feel about things are not mental illnesses that need psychiatric help. Nor do they always, or often need drug treatment. They are problems of adapting to a changing world and changes in your place in the world in which you live.

The book gives a few simple guidelines, and obviously you should seek help if depression is affecting work or family life, but there are other prompts to action:

- If people close to you say you should seek support then do so – too many people suffer alone
- If you are consistently waking more than an hour earlier than usual and are feeling low at that time

- If you are considering harming yourself or killing yourself, seek help immediately
- If your mood swings wildly up and down
- If you are having bizarre experiences such as hearing voices when no one is there

Depression occurring for the first time in midlife without an obvious cause such as a problem at work may be a result of the realisation that midlife has arrived. As I said earlier, this should not be regarded as the beginning of the end but it is certainly a time for reappraisal of where you want to take your life.

Anxiety is a normal response to uncertainty, and midlife is certainly full of uncertainty, but it should be regarded as a problem in two situations. The first is when anxiety occurs with no obvious external cause and starts to affect your ability to do your job or relate well to other family members. The second situation is where there is an obvious cause, for example financial problems or problems at work, but where the anxiety actually gets in the way of you solving the problem that is causing the anxiety. When you realise you have a problem and have to choose which option is best there is always an anxious period while you decide what to do and then wait to see if the result is what you planned. If, however, you become so anxious that you become paralysed and unable to take the decisions you need to take, then anxiety becomes a problem that has to be tackled. There are drugs to treat anxiety which do help the sufferer, the famous Librium, for example, but as with many mental health issues drug treatment should be taken carefully. There are good psychological techniques which you can learn not only to reduce your level of anxiety but also to prevent disabling anxiety striking again.

Midlife is a challenging time for the mind, which leads to problems. In your twenties, your teenage angst is receding and there is often a clear focus for the mind. The first years in your chosen career, or the development of a stable relationship (perhaps with marriage), provide a relatively stable set of activities for the mind to manage. In your thirties, things may get tougher – particularly if children have entered your life. But it is in midlife that the challenge for the mind becomes serious. Children leave home or change may happen at work (including dissatisfaction and boredom with a job that originally seemed ideal). Your relationship may also change during midlife. This may be only the psychological dimension or it may be complicated by a change in the sexual relationship and expectations of the partners.

It is therefore important to think how best to manage these challenges, and just as keeping fit physically reduces the risk of physical problems (and improves your mental well-being as a bonus), keeping mentally fit decreases the risk of mental problems and allows you to recover quickly if problems do develop. Obviously you can consult your GP about anxiety or depression but there are steps you can take yourself. Firstly you can understand what is happening and use the technique called cognitive behavioural therapy (CBT); you can find resources to help you with this in the Moodzone on NHS Choices.

The term cognitive behavioural therapy differentiates the treatment from drug therapy. Cognitive behavioural therapy is based on the concept that your thoughts, feelings and physical sensations are all interconnected, and that negative thoughts and feelings can trap you in a vicious cycle. The aim of CBT is to help you deal with all of your overwhelming problems in a more positive way by breaking them down into smaller, more manageable parts. The initial aim of CBT when it started was to simply offer an alternative to drug therapy based on the principle that if you change the way you think and behave you will change the way you feel.

CBT is now evolving from this simple model. If you change

how you think, you will change how you feel. It is highly rational and logical to recognise that some people need help in taking things less seriously and worrying less about the past and the future – these are things outside your control. There is now a type of cognitive therapy called MBCT: mindfulness-based cognitive therapy. It encourages you to learn mindfulness techniques to spend less time with your mind crowded with negative thoughts, and more with positive ones. There are plenty of opportunities for you to practise thinking better by yourself and practising mindfulness is one of them.

Mindfulness is described by the Mental Health Foundation as 'a mental state achieved by focusing one's awareness on the present moment, while calmly acknowledging and accepting feelings, thoughts, and bodily sensations'.

Here are some simple, easy-to-do tips on how to be more mindful:

- Take a couple of minutes to notice your breathing. Take long, deep breaths for five minutes a day to relax and gather your thoughts.
- Try something new. This doesn't have to be something complicated or extreme, it can just be sitting somewhere new in the office, or eating somewhere different for lunch.
- Name your thoughts and feelings when they appear, as this will develop your awareness.

Mental well-being is a health problem for which services and support can be delivered through the Internet. These are effective and are easy to access. The NHS Choices Moodzone contains not only information about mental health problems but also self-help tools which you can use to try to reduce the level of distress which is causing difficulty. For example, the section on depression contains information, a self-help technique supported by a podcast and advice on when and how urgently to seek help. Often, it is good to speak to someone and the Moodzone keeps an up-to-date list of all the mental health helplines, the telephone support services, mostly organised by charities. There are numerous charities and websites which are used to help combat stress.

1. Anxiety UK – This charity provides support if you've been diagnosed with an anxiety condition.
2. Bipolar UK – This is a charity helping people living with bipolar disorder (manic depression).
3. CALM – CALM is the Campaign Against Living Miserably, for men aged between 15 and 35.
4. Depression Alliance – This is a charity for sufferers of depression and it has a network of self-help groups.
5. Mental Health Foundation – The Foundation provides information and support for anyone with mental health problems or learning disabilities.
6. Mind – This important charity promotes the views and needs of people with mental health problems.
7. No Panic – This charity offers support for sufferers of panic attacks and obsessive compulsive disorder (OCD). It also offers a course to help overcome your phobia or OCD.
8. OCD Action – This provides support for people with obsessive compulsive disorder (OCD). It includes information on treatment and online resources.
9. OCD UK – This charity is run by people with OCD, for people with OCD.
10. PAPYRUS – The aim of this charity is to prevent suicides in young people.
11. Rethink Mental Illness – This is an important charity that provides support and advice for people living with mental illness.

12. Samaritans – The Samaritans provide confidential support for people experiencing feelings of distress or despair.
13. SANE – This charity offers support and carries out research into mental illness.

Part Two

Sleeping Better

Resources to help you sleep better	What's in it for you
Health Check	Questions about sleep are not routinely asked in the Health Check interview
One You	You are asked about how well you sleep in the How Are You quiz
Your annual review if you have a long-term condition like type 2 diabetes or high blood pressure	The person carrying out the review might not ask about sleep but you should bring it up if it is a problem that has developed after your condition has developed
NHS Choices	NHS Choices has a number of sections on how to sleep better, for example '10 tips to beat insomnia'
High-quality apps	Have a look at www.healthline.com for a review of sleep apps

Getting enough sleep is of great importance. But many midlifers find it difficult to achieve this – particularly those who are always busy. If you don't get enough sleep, not only will your quality of life be affected, but also your behaviour will change. Poor sleep is both a cause and a consequence of stress.

Tiredness

Tiredness is a heart-sinking problem, for doctors as well as for the sufferer. When the patient tells the doctor that he or she is tired the doctor has almost the whole of medicine to choose from as the cause. It could be anaemia resulting from cancer, it could be heart failure, it could be depression, it could be a neurological disease. The list is endless. Let's not forget that feeling exhausted is a common problem. Everyone, at some point in their life, will suffer from tiredness. Usually, there is nothing physically wrong. Most of the time, tiredness is linked with psychological problems such as stress.

Stress and anxiety, which cause insomnia, result in tiredness. Midlife is a time when stress can be at a premium, with the worries and strains of everyday life taking their toll on your mental well-being. Later on in this section, we will be looking at stress and how to tackle it to clear your mind.

Of course, there are physical causes which can cause tiredness. Being overweight or underweight, for example, can be a cause of tiredness. This is because your body is having to work much harder at everyday activities. If you are underweight especially, because you have less muscle, you work much harder. Take a look at the exercise section of this book to help tackle these issues. Tiredness is also linked with some lifestyle choices such as drinking too much alcohol, smoking and having a bad diet.

So, what can the doctor do? Not much, except advise the person who is tired to read this book.

To tackle tiredness, here is what I suggest:

- Get a little fitter
- Lose weight, intentionally
- Take action to reduce the stress reaction and become more positive
- Cut down on alcohol and drugs
- Take action to sleep longer and better

Although the amount of sleep people need varies from one person to another, it is sensible to have at least seven hours' sleep a night for at least five nights a week. For some lucky people this is what they get without effort, but many people find difficulty in getting off to sleep or wake in the night and lie awake for hours. We now understand the science of sleep better and we appreciate the need for sleep. There is no point in thinking, 'Oh, Mr and Mrs X manage on five hours of sleep a night, so I must be able to do it.' You are different from everyone else and your brain needs good-quality sleep. It may be that you need more sleep, not less, as you approach midlife. Some of the problems that people put down to 'old age' are simply due to lack of sleep.

The Science of Sleep

The scientific study of sleep has advanced greatly in the last decade, in part because of the awareness of the problem of sleep apnoea. In sleep apnoea, people (particularly those with respiratory problems) frequently stop breathing for a few seconds numerous times during the night, which obviously affects the quality of their sleep.

What you want to have is REM sleep, the letters REM standing for Rapid Eye Movement. NREM stands for Non-Rapid Eye Movement sleep, being further subdivided into N1, N2 and N3 stages, and you pass through the stages of REM, N1, N2 and N3 several times a night. REM sleep is when you dream and it is also the time when the key hormones – testosterone and oestrogen – are released into your bloodstream. The REM and NREM sleep alternate throughout the night but the latter half of the night is when REM dominates. For this reason, wrenching yourself from sleep with an alarm clock has a disruptive effect on the potential benefit of a good night's sleep. This is not, of course, a reason to sleep as long as you want; it is a reason to get to bed early and calmly prepared for a good night's sleep!

However, the analysis of sleep problems and their treatment is relatively simple and is based on studies of how people develop and solve sleeping problems rather than studies of the brain. There are five causes of sleep problems:

- your brain
- your mind
- your environment
- your body
- your behaviour

Each one of these has an effect on your sleeping pattern and routine. Now, let's take a look at each problem and what can be done to change that, starting with the brain. Chemicals in the brain can cause sleep problems, particularly caffeine, but many prescribed medicines have sleep problems as one of their side effects. So too do some recreational drugs such as alcohol. Remember, the older your brain is the more sensitive it becomes to the effects of chemicals. Usually 'sleeping difficulties' are just listed as one possible side effect in very small print in the leaflet in the box in which your tablets arrive, but if sleep problems develop after starting new medication ask your pharmacist for advice.

As for caffeine, which is in tea as well as coffee, it stimulates the brain and keeps you awake. It is essential to cut out caffeine after 6pm if you have difficulty in getting off to sleep. Some people find they have to stop drinking tea or coffee much earlier than 6pm. If you are on prescribed medicines ask your pharmacist if they could be causing sleeping difficulty. If they say yes, you may want to discuss changing your medicines with your doctor.

Even if your brain is not affected by caffeine or other drugs, your mind can keep you awake. Anxiety is a root cause of sleeping difficulties, as is depression. People who are anxious often find it difficult to get to sleep, people who are depressed may wake up early and, of course, some people are both anxious and depressed.

The cognitive function of the mind is to do with thinking and planning, and therefore worrying, and for many people what keeps them awake is worry. Their mind goes over and over certain issues – 'Should I take that job offer?', 'How are we going to pay the bills next month?', 'Why does our relationship feel strained?' These are examples of the types of thinking that keep people awake at night. Sleep problems are a very common feature of stress, and stress is our response to a challenge in the environment in which we live.

Even if you cannot sort out the financial or work problems that are the cause of the stress, which in turn is the cause of your sleeping problems, there are steps you can take. You can use some of the relaxation techniques described at the end of this chapter every evening before you go to bed to develop your pre-sleep routine.

For some people, sleeping pills are the answer. But whilst sleeping pills can help you in the short term, they are not the answer to help you improve your quality of sleep. It is important that, if taking sleeping pills, they do not become habit-forming. They should be a short-term solution whilst you change your lifestyle and habits. Alongside the techniques described above, the NHS Choices website contains good information for people with insomnia – all of which are much better than sleeping pills.

The environment in which you live has both physical and social challenges. Physical activity and staying active will always make you sleep better. But, challenges in your social environment can often lead to stress and disrupt your sleeping patterns. Think of the challenges that people face in midlife, often more than one:

- Work, particularly shift work
- Children, either young children who wake early or, even worse, teenagers who come in late
- Relationship difficulties
- Housing and financial problems

The first step, of course, is to solve the underlying problem, which may be very difficult, or impossible. Of the common problems listed above, perhaps the one that is most amenable to action is difficulty with a relationship. Housing and finance problems are difficult to overcome and problems at work usually relate to people over whom you have little control, namely the boss. However, difficulties with your partner are within your power to influence.

The second step is to reduce the impact of the stress reaction which stimulates the brain just when you are trying to sleep. But remember, it is not possible to blame stress alone for poor sleep and some people sleep badly even if they are not stressed. The problem may be in the way you try to get to sleep.

One environmental factor that often gets overlooked is your mattress. It is not an inexpensive item but you need to ask yourself if your mattress could be better. Mattresses age just like human beings and your mattress may just not be up to the job any longer. There is no rule about how hard or soft a mattress should be, it has to be right for you and if you are a couple a zipped pair of single mattresses, one hard and the other soft, may be the answer.

People with long-term conditions such as arthritis often have sleep disturbance as a direct consequence of the symptoms caused by the disease, notably pain. Getting fitter will help your sleep but most experts advise against vigorous exercise before you try to get to sleep. The types of exercise designed to promote suppleness can help people sleep better, in part because these types of exercise often focus on relaxation of the mind as well as increasing the suppleness of the body, so a short ritual of stretching for five minutes before you get into bed may help. For some people itching is a cause of disturbed sleep and a generous application of aqueous cream is very effective in reducing that problem.

'Bedtime' is one of the first words we learn and there is

evidence that a regular bedtime helps children get off to sleep, often accompanied by a ritual, the story, the kiss and a statement such as 'love you'. When we are grown-ups, we have the freedom to decide when to go to bed. Some people can go to bed at any time and drift off quickly but for others a failure to have a regular routine, including a regular bedtime, is the principal cause of their sleep problems.

If you sleep at least seven hours at least five nights a week and don't feel tired, you don't have a problem. If, on the other hand, you feel you have a problem, or tell other people you have insomnia, you should try to tackle the problem by yourself before going to the GP seeking a sleeping pill, because reliance on sleeping pills for the long term is not a good idea – all medicines have side effects and can do harm as well as good. Try to identify the cause or causes of your sleep problem.

Possible cause	Important for you
In your brain, e.g. caffeine after 6pm or possible side effects of prescribed medicines	
In your body, e.g. painful joints or grumbling tummy pains	
In your mind, e.g. anxiety, depression, worrying or stress	
In your environment, e.g. noisy children, a cold bed	
In your behaviour, e.g. watching exciting films just before you go to bed	

There is no quick fix for long-term sleep problems but, depending on your analysis of the causes of your problems, there are things you can do. You will have to stick with your plan for at least a month and then, if necessary, review it and adjust it again to find the formula for good sleep for the rest of your life.

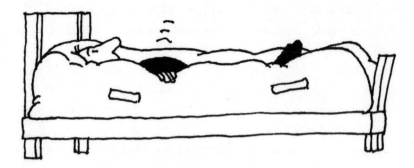

Firstly, make sure that your home environment does not keep you awake.

- Maintain a comfortable sleeping environment that's not too hot or cold. Find the temperature that suits you.
- Noise can also be a great distractor for sleep. Earplugs or soothing music will dampen external sounds and give you a better chance of sleep.
- Lower the light levels around your home at a certain time. Lower light levels can induce sleep by signalling to your brain to produce melatonin – the hormone that helps you sleep.
- Turn off TVs, computers and other devices (like tablets or phones) at least an hour before bed.

Secondly, try to develop a routine.

- Establish fixed times for going to bed and waking up.
- Put aside work, difficult decisions or upcoming deadlines at least two hours before you sleep. Instead, occupy your mind by reading, listening to music or taking a bath.
- Make a list of things that you need to achieve the next day.

- Drink a warm caffeine-free drink, such as peppermint or camomile tea, before you sleep.
- Clean your teeth and floss for five minutes.

Thirdly, you should try to avoid the following:

- Try not to eat heavy or spicy foods before you sleep as they can overload your digestive system.
- Avoid nicotine and alcohol late at night. Nicotine acts as a stimulant and tobacco can keep you from falling asleep. Alcohol, on the other hand, may help to initially induce sleep, but once the effects have worn off, you will be awake many times throughout the night.
- Don't listen to or watch discussion programmes that will annoy you.

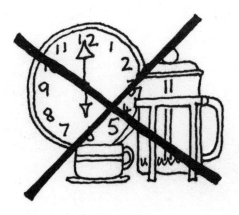

Healthy sleep habits can have a positive effect on your quality of life and health. Reducing stress and improving sleep will give your body more energy and will help you focus on the task ahead. You will feel motivated to get fitter. Now, let's take a look at how we can do that.

Part Three

Getting Fit

Resources on getting fitter	What's in it for you
Health Check	You will be asked about your levels of physical activity
One You	The How Are You quiz asks (1) how many minutes a day you spend on activities that change your breathing, for example brisk walking (2) how many minutes a day you spend on activities that keep your muscles and bones strong
Your annual review if you have a long-term condition like type 2 diabetes or high blood pressure	If there is time you may be given advice about the need to keep active or get more active to counteract the effects of many long-term conditions on physical activity. However there is often insufficient time because so much of the time is taken up discussing the drugs you are on
NHS Choices	• The 10,000 steps challenge gives information about the benefits of walking, but don't be put off by the 10,000 target. If you commute in a car or bus to a desk job you will find it difficult to hit the 10,000 target, no matter how hard you try. A better approach, now being promoted by experts, is to aim to increase your walking by 3,000 steps and, remembering that 1,000 steps takes ten minutes, try to fit first one, then two, then three ten-minute sessions of brisk walking into your day

(continued)

Resources on getting fitter	What's in it for you
	• For those people who want to do more, there is the great Couch to 5K challenge, which encourages people to try to change gear and start running, and this is available as an app on the One You website. For those people who can run 5k there is the 5K+ challenge with advice on how to improve your stamina even more, and enjoy it while you do. You can also join the wonderful parkrun movement
High-quality apps	Try www.mapmywalk.com/app and the One You Couch to 5K app

The excellent survey of physical activity carried out by the British Heart Foundation and the University of Oxford revealed some worrying trends in 2015:

• People in midlife are less active than people in their thirties.
• People in their forties and fifties are more active than people in their sixties.
• People in midlife spend increased amounts of time every day and every week in that very dangerous activity: sitting down.

The drop in physical activity between the ages of 30 and 60 leads to a dramatic drop in health. If you are in your forties or fifties, this is what you should be aiming for:

1. Adults should aim to be active daily. Over a week, activity should add up to at least 150 minutes (2.5 hours) of moderate-intensity activity in bouts of 10 minutes or more – one way to approach this is to do 30 minutes on at least 5 days a week.

2. Alternatively, comparable benefits can be achieved through 75 minutes of vigorous-intensity activity spread across the week or a combination of moderate and vigorous activity.
3. Adults should also undertake physical activity to improve muscle strength on at least 2 days a week.
4. All adults should minimise the amount of time spent being sedentary (sitting) for extended periods.

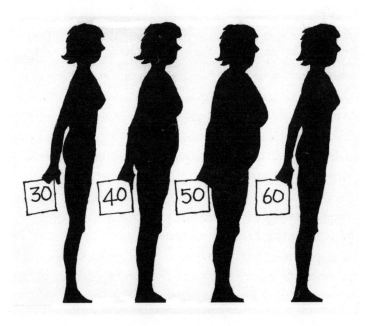

How fit are you?

If you look at ten people in their forties or fifties, whilst they are sitting down, you might be able to guess how fit they are. But sometimes people who look fit are actually very *unfit*. To judge how fit people are you have to give them some work to do, as a test. You could ask them to walk up to the fourth floor without stopping or do 50 press-ups, and when they had done the test you could soon judge who was fit and who was not. The very fit would not have turned a hair, the quite fit would be a little out of breath and the least fit would be most distressed and would take longest to recover; the very unfit ones might not even complete the test.

In the exercise part of the How Are You quiz, the first question simply asks how much exercise that 'makes you breathe harder . . . e.g. fast walking, cycling, sport' you get every day. Second, you are asked 'How much strengthening activity do you do? For example weights, sit-ups, yoga, carrying heavy shopping, digging the garden'. For each question, you are asked how many minutes you spend each day on activities that will either increase your stamina or your strength.

As you get older, the ability to do things decreases, but not by much if you keep fit. In his book *Fast After 50,* Joe Friel, a triathlete himself who is now over 70, demonstrates how the performance of athletes and cyclists does not decline by much until the age of 80. Also, he points out that even athletes in their fifties training for a triathlon are probably not doing it with the same crazy intensity as they did in their thirties, because their attitude to training has changed. So the difference in performance between 30-year-old athletes and 50-year-old athletes is not due to ageing alone but to ageing plus a change in attitude.

Ageing, however, results not only in a loss of ability; it results in a loss of resilience. This means that the older you are, the quicker you lose fitness and the slower you regain the loss of ability. If a 20-year-old has to be immobile for a month, they will lose fitness, but a 50-year-old immobilised for the same time will lose more and take longer to get it back.

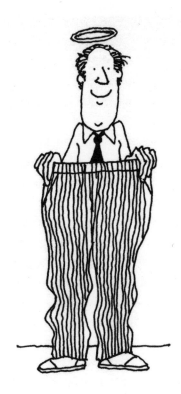

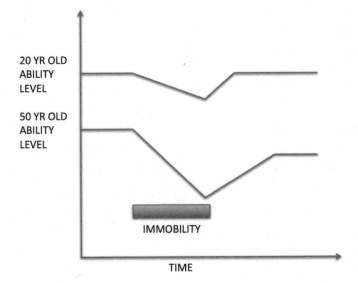

How inactive are you?

It's no surprise that people are much less active these days. Whilst technology has made our lives easier, it has also hindered our exercise.

We use public transport or, even worse, our cars to get to work, rather than walking or cycling. We sit for hours in front of the TV or computer at home. We move around less and use less energy as desk working increases and housework becomes less physical and, as a result, we're becoming obese. It has been the decline in energy expenditure rather than an increase in energy intake that has led to the epidemic of obesity. Inactivity has been described as a 'silent killer'. Sitting or lying down for long periods is bad for your health. It is vitally important that you begin to raise your activity levels. In addition to the decrease in energy use over time there is a decrease in energy use as we grow older. Research published by the British Heart Foundation shows that people aged 60 sit for an hour more every day than people aged 40. This has nothing to do with ageing; it is just a gradual change in lifestyle.

People who have been on their feet for four hours or more a day are certainly entitled to flop on a sofa in the evening, but people who have been sitting for eight hours at a desk, with commuting on top, need to be aware that the tiredness they feel is the result of sitting. It needs to be countered by activity, and that does not mean going to the gym but an hour or two painting the spare room or ironing or tidying a cupboard! New research suggests that even if you walk or run for 150 minutes a week you are still at increased risk of poor health if you sit for long periods at work or at home. The TV, the computer screen and the sofa are all major threats to health.

Sitting at home also presents its challenges. Matt Rudd wrote a powerful attack on sofas in the *Sunday Times* of 24 April 2016:

> Sofa manufacturers are in an arms race with our bottoms. The bigger our bottoms, the bigger and softer are the sofas that have to support them. The bigger and softer, the bigger our bottoms become . . . so if I really loved my family, I'd get rid of the sofa and replace it with a standing space. Ironically my family won't stand for that.

So, we need to avoid sitting. An hour a day of sitting rather than standing is 420 calories less used every week (nearly 22,000 less in a year), which is equivalent to about 7 pounds (3 kilos) of fat. Let's get the equation right:

> 1 extra hour a day sitting = 7 pounds (3 kilos) more fat by the end of a year

Work has changed in the last 50 years, and thank goodness for that. For many people, however, work means sitting down for six or eight hours a day and this increases the risk of vascular diseases such as stroke, heart disease and type 2

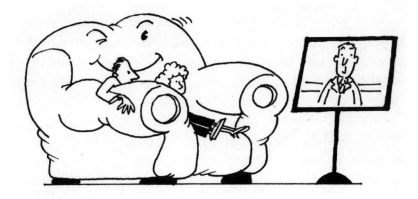

diabetes, which some campaigners say should now be renamed 'walking deficiency syndrome' or 'hyper-sitting syndrome'.

Naturally, previous generations were much more active than we are today. The work they did (such as manual labour) demanded more physical activity. Today, many of our jobs require sitting down which in turn makes us lazier and less healthy. The environment that we are in is proving to be the biggest challenge. By moving less, you are putting your health at a risk of many chronic diseases such as heart disease, stroke, weight gain, type 2 diabetes and obesity. Daniel Lieberman, a Harvard professor, calls these 'mismatch diseases'. He argues that these diseases are caused by the fact that we have bodies which evolved to survive in an environment that required us to roam and wander the plains to find food.

When we see Bear Grylls in the wild, roaming extreme places and struggling to survive, it looks as though he is in a dangerous environment – the weather, the lack of food, the lack of human contact. But in fact, the Stone Age environment and lifestyle, running about in the fresh air looking for food, was good for your health – if you could scrape together a diet of meat and vegetables. Obesity and immobility were not problems then. Our environment has changed and we have as well. It's time to tackle the new urban environment and get moving.

Sitting uses one calorie per minute, while standing uses two calories per minute, and although the difference sounds small, it all adds up. If you were to stand for even two of the eight hours daily for a year, that would be the equivalent to the energy used to run about 15 marathons.

You don't need to worry about asking your boss for a £1,000 standing desk or, if you are the boss, buying standing desks for everyone (although these desks are cool, especially the ones that have a treadmill as well). All you need is either to find a surface of the right height – a four-drawer filing cabinet for taller people, and a three-drawer one for the shorter – or buy a plastic storage box of the right depth from an office equipment supplier to turn upside down on your desk. You can also buy very simple lecterns to put the paper you are reading or writing on at the right height for your eyes and hands.

There are numerous ways that you can keep fit at the workplace. Here is a brief list of the things that you or your team can do:

- Leave your desk at lunch time for at least ten minutes of walking.
- Use the stairs rather than the lift. There's a great system for encouraging the use of stairs with a free app for workers, a simple way of recording the number of steps climbed and, beside every lift, a sign and a 2D barcode that the app can read. Have a look at www.stepjockey.com.
- Stand and stretch every hour (if at a keyboard).
- Get a Pilates or tai chi teacher to come in once a month to teach and reinforce the need for stretching and good posture.
- Buy some low-cost weights: 3kg dumb-bells, 5kg kettle-bells, and a 10kg bar.
- Put a hanging bar in a doorway.

As well as increasing the risk of major problems such as type 2 diabetes, sitting is bad for the neck, shoulders and spine. Some of the damage can be minimised by stretching your shoulders, upper limbs, neck and spine before you attack the keyboard, and also periodically throughout the day.

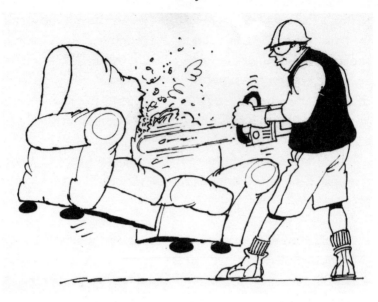

How much can getting fitter reduce your risk?

Whatever your age, there is strong scientific evidence that being physically active can lead to a healthier and happier life. You will be less likely to develop many of the common diseases – stroke, type 2 diabetes, depression, heart disease, dementia and even some cancers. Physical activity can also boost self-esteem, sleep quality and energy.

Exercise is the miracle cure we've always had. But for too long, we've neglected to take our recommended dose. Doctors are now prescribing walking and other forms of physical activity, rather than just providing pills and medicine.

You may not think about, or want to think about, the future very much but you are on a journey and getting fitter in midlife gives you a much better chance of enjoying yourself well into old age. Here are a few health benefits for those that do regular physical activity:

- up to a 35% lower risk of coronary heart disease and stroke
- up to a 50% lower risk of type 2 diabetes
- up to a 50% lower risk of colon cancer
- up to a 20% lower risk of breast cancer
- up to a 30% lower risk of early death
- up to an 83% lower risk of osteoarthritis
- up to a 68% lower risk of hip fracture
- up to a 30% lower risk of depression
- up to a 30% lower risk of dementia

By getting fitter in your midlife, you will regain the ability and physical level you had when you were 30. If you keep fit and keep training, then you will never drop below the line at which you become very dependent on others. The journey starts here.

As I have mentioned, adults should be active daily and aim to achieve at least 150 minutes of physical activity over a week. For any type of activity to benefit you and your health, you need to be moving quickly enough to raise your heart rate, breathe faster and feel warmer. Physical fitness has four aspects and they all begin with the letter S:

- Strength
- Suppleness
- Stamina
- Skill

Improving your strength and suppleness

Middle-aged people are, on average, weaker than younger people. But this loss of strength is not just because of age. No, this loss of strength is also due to inactivity. The good news for people who are over 40 is that if they start doing regular, focused exercise they can dramatically improve their strength and regain lost power – with power being the ability of muscles to move quickly when needed.

Your strength is determined by your muscles, the red stuff in a leg of lamb; your suppleness is determined by your ligaments and tendons, the white stuff in a leg of lamb. Tendons join muscle to bone and ligaments join bone to bone.

The white stuff is made up of two chemicals – collagen and elastin – and one of the effects of ageing is the reduction of the amount of elastin relative to the amount of collagen. However, most of the loss of suppleness, the stiffness that develops as we grow older, is not the result of this change in the chemistry but of the inactivity that most of us have to put up with from about the age of 20 on.

In your forties and fifties, loss of suppleness does not have the type of major disabling consequences that it can have in your seventies. However, most people in their fifties will reach their seventies, and will still want to be able to put on their tights or tie their shoelaces, so tackling loss of suppleness in your fifties is a good insurance policy. There are immediate benefits from taking steps to improve your suppleness in your fifties because many of the aches and pains in your neck, back, shoulders and hips can be both prevented and improved by simple stretching exercises.

The NHS Choices Strength and Flex plan is a five-week plan consisting of equipment-free exercises designed to improve your strength and flexibility. The workout instructions are easy to follow and ensure that you are exercising correctly and at the right pace. The great thing about this plan is that you can do these full body workouts wherever and whenever is most convenient for you. Regular focused exercise can be called training, and although the term training is usually associated with participation in a particular sport, why not think of yourself as being in training – it also helps you refuse that doughnut or lunchtime drink.

But remember, it's not just for five weeks but for five decades. In addition to the Strength and Flex plan, NHS Choices website has a number of excellent suppleness videos. Remember too that although some people develop a specific form of joint disease called rheumatoid arthritis which needs expert and early medical treatment, most people with stiff and painful joints have other problems, some of which come from the smooth joint surface wearing out but all of which are aggravated by our modern lifestyle. Arthritis Research, the main charity, is clear: 'Your body is designed to move and not doing so can harm the tissues in and around your joints. Many people are afraid to exercise because they believe that it damages their joints. But keeping active will help to keep your joints supple and reduce pain.'

You can do activities that strengthen your muscles on the same day or on different days as your aerobic activity – whatever's best for you. Muscle-strengthening exercises are not an aerobic activity, so you'll need to do them in addition to your 150 minutes of aerobic activity. Some vigorous activities count as both an aerobic activity and a muscle-strengthening activity.

Examples include:

- circuit training
- aerobics
- running
- football
- rugby
- netball
- hockey

The How Are You and Health Check quizzes will ask how active you are but the activity is not always as beneficial as it could be, and you need to be sure you are focusing on all aspects of fitness, including strength. It may be, of course, that you get enough muscle training at work. How would you describe your work, or your life at home if you are not in paid employment?

1	Using all your muscles all the time	
2	Using all your muscles several hours a day, for example lifting boxes or cases	
3	Using your muscles for a short time some days	
4	Sitting at a desk or console all day	

If you are in Group 1 or Group 2 you are probably getting enough strength training but you may need to concentrate on suppleness to prevent back or shoulder problems. If you are in Group 3 or Group 4, you need to start a daily training routine. You need to do strengthening exercises every day and if you can go somewhere to lift heavy weights, so much the better.

You need to build up the muscles in your chest, upper limbs and lower limbs and the core muscles of your back and abdomen. The three main muscle groups helped by weights are the chest, the upper limbs and lower limbs. Don't try to strengthen your spine by weightlifting without a coach; do that with the floor exercises recommended in your ten-minute daily workout.

The additional benefit of muscle strengthening is that the same exercises strengthen your bones and greater bone strength is a very important part of planning for future health, particularly for women because it will reduce the risk of fractures.

Here are three exercises you can do as part of your daily ten minutes of strength and suppleness training, using the weight of your own body, without the need for any equipment.

- For the upper limbs remember the classic press-up. A man aged 50 should be able to do 50 press-ups, maybe not immediately but after three months' training it will be possible.

- For the core muscles there are three exercises that will produce a flat stomach and will be the foundation of a six-pack.
    - Lie flat on your back, legs straight, then lift the heels 6 inches off the ground, open them to shoulder width, then criss-cross them 60 times.
    - Then roll over onto your front, hands behind the back of your head, and lift your forehead off the floor, arching your back. Repeat five times, counting slowly to ten at the top of each lift.
    - Side Plank: Rest on one elbow and forearm, facing to the side, and keep your body in a straight line. Hold for 30 seconds then turn to face the other way and repeat. Complete the entire cycle twice.
- For the lower limbs just do squats: stand with your feet slightly apart and bend your knees till you are sitting on an invisible chair. Do ten squats then do some stretching and do 80, in eight sets of ten, with stretching between each set.

Utilising your body weight is a good place to start the process of getting stronger. Alongside the exercises above, which require no equipment, there is kit available to help you increase your strength:

- **Resistance bands** – These are made of elastic and are very good for arms and shoulders. They come in different strengths, so start with a medium-strength band. If it is too difficult, grasp it with your hands further apart; if it is too easy, grasp it with your hands closer together. They are not expensive and you can even find them in pound shops. Resistance bands are sometimes easy but of course two or three can be used together for added strength and difficulty.

- **Hand weights** – These come in pairs, one for each hand. There are two types, dumb-bells with a grip in the middle or kettle-bells with a little handle on top. There is not much to choose between the two. A 50-year-old woman should be able to handle the 3kg pair, a man 5kg, although many women are stronger than some men. Weights are good for both upper and lower limbs; use them for your squats. These weights increase the impact of your daily dozen but can be used at other times. Leave them by the television and use them every ad break! Weights are particularly important for women, so that they can strengthen their bones and reduce the risk of fractures in the long term.

- **Big weights** – These are on a simple bar and can be 20kg, 30kg or more. At least twice a week it is good to use big weights but they are obviously more expensive, and unless you have a garage or shed, they consume a bit of space. You can use them in a gym and it is good to get some instruction on how to use them without harming your back. If you can, club together and buy a set for the office.

It is not only your muscles that benefit from this type of training, it also helps your bones stay strong because, unlike machines, bones get stronger with repeated use and weaken with inactivity.

Both strength and suppleness will be improved by these routines (among hundreds of other options) but there are two other S's in fitness – skill and stamina. In your fifties you might not need to worry too much about losing skill but you do need to take action to maintain and improve your stamina.

Improving your stamina

Stamina is your ability to sustain prolonged physical activity (or mental activity) and is the clearest indicator to evaluate your health and fitness level. It is also a key component in achieving improved fitness levels and decreasing heart problems.

Most people start to lose stamina in their early twenties when they get a car, get a job that involves sitting and give up sport.

So, how active are you?

How do you get to work?		Points
	Walk or cycle	3
	Public transport	2
	Car	1

At work, are you:		Points
	On your feet all the time?	3
	Sitting about half the time?	2
	Sitting all of the time?	1

How do you spend your evening?		Points
	On the go doing things most of the time	3
	Sitting, e.g. watching TV, for less than two hours	2
	Sitting, e.g. watching TV, for more than two hours	1

Now add up your score.

Score	Meaning
7, 8 or 9	Your lifestyle is healthy and if you are on your feet all day you deserve a seat in the evening. However, you should try our walking programme or take other exercise to get you breathless.
4, 5 or 6	You definitely need to increase the amount of time you take doing aerobic exercise: that is, exercise that makes you breathless.
3	You definitely need to build aerobic exercise into your week. In your fifties you don't need to worry about your heart unless there is heart disease in your family, but you need to get going. It may be that your weight is part of the problem or you may be a smoker, so you need to tackle those underlying problems, but you also need to take steps, lots of them, to get fitter.

If you want a quick check of your stamina, take the stairs and not the lift to go up four floors and then answer the question below.

How breathless were you on the fourth floor?	Not breathless at all	
	A bit breathless but did not have to stop	
	Had to stop and get my breath back	

If you were not breathless at all, well done, but don't get complacent. If you were breathless, then you definitely need to take action. You will feel better within a month and you will get a big pay-off in your sixties and seventies if you start increasing your stamina now. Of course if you have bronchitis, or chronic obstructive pulmonary disease (COPD) as it is now called, then you will become breathless more easily. COPD results from cigarette smoking or, increasingly, air pollution and is a common condition which needs good treatment and a good exercise programme to close the fitness gap, as the British Lung Foundation clearly describes.

Improving your skill

The fourth aspect of physical fitness beginning with the letter 'S' is skill.

Taking up a sport in your forties will greatly benefit your balance and hand-eye coordination. We have already looked at various options, but there are many other activities that you can take up to increase your skill. Furthermore, you could take up a new active hobby like Latin American dancing or step aerobics on your birthday, or as a birthday present, setting a trend for other birthdays at each of which you should also take up something new, or get lessons and training to do whatever you enjoy even more, such as swimming.

Designing your 4S fitness plan

It is increasingly clear, however, that getting physically fitter has a number of other benefits, namely:

- preventing and reducing depression
- reducing the feelings of stress
- improving sleep
- reducing the risk of dementia

The exercises for strength, stamina, suppleness and skill have been described in this way to help you get your mind round the different aspects of fitness that you need to think about and work on every day. However, the body is not divided into separate systems for skill or suppleness or stamina or strength. All these things rely on different bits of the body and different systems working together. The best plan is to focus on your overall risk. There is little point in improving your diet but not increasing the amount of exercise that you do, or the other way round. You have to see the whole picture and that's where the One You quiz helps. This principle applies to your health in general and to your fitness. The best exercise is exercise that tests all four aspects of fitness, for example ten little squat jumps, preferably with a 1kg or 3kg weight in each hand, or ten burpees (squat thrust).

Whilst it is important to keep active and develop an exercise plan, it is also important to think about your body whilst you are resting. By the age of 40, too many people, particularly those who spend their working life looking at a computer screen, have started to develop a bad posture. If you were to ask people to draw an image of old age it would be the forward stoop, head poked out like a tortoise, that you can still see on old road signs. This is due to spinal disease in only a very small number of people. In almost everyone it is the result of bad habits when sitting, standing or walking, so here is what to do.

At least once a day:

- Lie flat on the floor on your back with arms stretched out, and the backs of your hands on the ground. Now slide your arms upwards as far as you can, keeping elbows and hands on the carpet. Do this ten times. If you can't do this in your workplace, do this exercise instead:
  - Stand facing a corner, one foot in front of the other.
  - Place one hand on each wall at shoulder height, arms straight.
  - Keeping your spine straight, bend your elbows and touch (or nearly touch) the corner with your forehead.

- Now hold your arms at shoulder height with elbows bent, and then try to touch your elbows behind your back – don't worry, no one can, but try to stretch your chest muscles ten times.
- Now wrap each arm across your chest so that your right-hand fingertips reach round your left arm and try to touch your spine – don't worry, no one can, but stretch ten times.

Do these exercises at least once a day. If you are driving or sitting all day, try to do the exercises three times a day – get the whole office moving.

In addition:

- Never stand with your arms folded – it pulls the spine forward.
- Imagine how you look and use mirrors or shop windows to give you a glimpse of yourself two or three times a day.
- Stand as often and as long as you can instead of peering tortoise-like at the computer screen.
- Imagine the crown of your head is attached to a string, and make sure the crown and not the forehead is your highest point.
- Beware of peering at your phone as you walk. Every inch your head is ahead of the true vertical line increases the weight your neck muscles have to hold by ten pounds (about 4.5kg) and if you do it for long enough, often enough, your head will be permanently poking forward, like a tortoise.

There are practitioners who have the skills to help you when some problem of overuse and misuse occurs, usually pains in the neck, shoulders and back. Even more importantly, they can help you learn how to prevent a recurrence of your current problem and the other problems that arise from that dangerous combination of commuting, deskwork, computing and – last but not least – the TV and the sofa.

Getting fitter through walking

Walking is the simplest and best form of exercise to increase your stamina and reduce your stress too. If you spend half or all of the working day sitting, and have to drive to and from work, try to build time for walking into your life.

The aim should be an *extra* 150 minutes of brisk walking each week. In midlife you are busy, so an extra 30 minutes every weekday might seem a big ask, but you do need to do it, especially if you scored six or less in the test above. So here is what you could do:

- Get to your workplace with time for a ten-minute walk before you start work, or just park ten minutes further away. When you arrive at your workplace, avoid the lift. Taking the stairs every day will help improve your stamina.
- Use your lunchtime as a time to walk; ask others to join you – they will. You can walk for a charity using a step counter. The walking apps are accurate enough but you may want to buy, or ask for as a present, a Fitbit or similar piece of kit.
- An additional benefit of the lunchtime walk is that the sunlight (which is always there except on the darkest days) gives your vitamin D a boost.*

---

* Vitamin D deficiency is now a serious problem which carries its own risks, and women in particular should make sure that they get enough calcium from semi-skimmed (or skimmed) milk and take 25µg of vitamin D a day if sunlight is in short supply.

- Take your final ten-minute walk in the evening, perhaps with your partner.

This is just one example of how you can easily and quickly improve your stamina. There are many other ways that you can get fitter, so find whatever works for you.

Remember:

> 10 minutes = 1,000 steps = 40 calories = 1 biscuit
> 10 minutes daily, 5 days a week for a year = 10 pounds of fat
> Get your pulse up 150 minutes a week
> Get breathless 75 minutes a week

Walking does not mean sauntering, ambling, strolling or stopping every two minutes to check your phone. You should walk briskly enough to notice that your breathing rate has increased, but not so fast that you struggle to talk. Your ten-minute walks should be taken at a brisk pace, but you should still be able to make a mobile-phone call or converse with the person walking with you, and these are good ways to build walking into your work. If you have the freedom to leave the office when you have a phone call or when you have a one-to-one meeting, do them whilst walking.

In recent years, the Ramblers (a long-established charity) has been developing and changing its role in the walking world. It will still campaign for access to the countryside but it is also promoting the benefits of walking as the single best form of exercise, and it is aiming at recruiting younger people not only to walk but also to create trails and walks in both the countryside and cities.

Finally, although golf has been called 'a good walk spoiled', a round of golf, without a buggy, can sometimes use more energy than a game of rugby.

Getting fitter through running and high-intensity training

It is 8.59 on Saturday morning, any Saturday morning, and in about 100,000 places round the world people line up to start their parkrun. This is an astounding health service, started by volunteers in Bushy Park in Teddington and still organised by volunteers. There is a great, clear website which you can join at www.parkrun.com and you can record your times there (or not, if you prefer not to).

The Couch to 5K app is a great way to start your journey to better health but what happens when you can run 5K? One option is to join a running club but they can look fairly terrifying, although they are friendly and welcoming. The running club is for people with their eyes on a half marathon or marathon. The parkrun is for people who want to run (or even walk and run) 5K in the company of friends or who just like running with others who are primarily encouraging rather than competitive. In a parkrun 'it doesn't matter how fast you go' and there is a 2K junior event for children.

There has always been a huge interest in running and this is a good way to get breathless. There isn't a better time to get a move on and get breathless. Real breathlessness, the sort that leaves you unable to talk and able only to stand with your hands on your knees till you recover, is good for you. The number of people participating in 5K, 10K, half marathons, marathons and ultramarathons has increased dramatically in recent years and by using the NHS Choices Couch to 5k programme almost everyone in midlife could do 5K.

However, if you don't have time to go running, or are embarrassed to be seen running, then you might want to choose another form of training – high-intensity training (HIT). HIT is a form of training whereby you repeat a certain number of exercises as fast as you can, flat out. This spikes your metabolism and builds muscle quickly. Unlike running, or other exercises, HIT burns calories during the workout as well as afterwards. If you repeat the same sets of exercises, but pause to regain your breath in between, this is called high-intensity interval training (HIIT). An example, which you can try at home, would be:

- 30 seconds: High knees
- 30 seconds: Squats
- 30 seconds: Basic burpees
- 30 seconds: Jumping jacks

You can increase the time you spend on each exercise to increase the difficulty. Remember, the most important thing is to raise your heart rate.

If you are an avid runner, try introducing HIIT to your daily run:

- 30 seconds: Sprint
- 15 seconds: Recover
- Repeat 1–2 times
- Continue regular run
- 30 seconds: Sprint
- 15 seconds: Recover
- Repeat 1–2 times

There are different ways to train and work out – from endurance training to marathon training, triathlon training to high-intensity interval training. Obviously the type of activity depends on your end goal, but high-intensity interval training is the best. Not only does it raise your heart rate and leave you breathless, but it has the advantage that it need not take three hours (or even one) to complete. Some of the programmes are so effective, they can even be completed in your lunch hour. The point of HIIT is that it is 'high-intensity' in name and nature. You might not be able to keep it up for more than a few minutes, or even a whole minute, but you can give it your best shot. As Joe Friel says, 'There may well be some good excuses for not training intensely, but age isn't one of them.'

Now, let's look at the other programmes recommended by the NHS that will leave you in a state of breathlessness:

- playing sport competitively
- swimming – swim non-stop for ten minutes
- running – you can run in one long burst or, like the HIIT training, you can try 'interval' running, but for efficient breathlessness interval running is best
- cycling is a good way of getting breathless but remember that cycling is the most efficient form of travel and it is all too easy to freewheel and admire the scenery

Getting fitter through competitive sports

Sport is too often associated with youth. Yes, more people play sport when they are younger, but this isn't due to their age. Instead, participation in sport dips when your time becomes more important – you work, you get married, you have children. All of these reduce your opportunity to get involved with a sport and as a result, when you reach 40, you think you're 'past it'.

Sport England are now recognising the importance and relevance of sport to people over 40. Many sports have been trying to increase the participation of people over the age of 40 for years. The League of Veteran Racing Cyclists organises races for people in their forties, as well as people in their sixties. Veteran leagues are popping

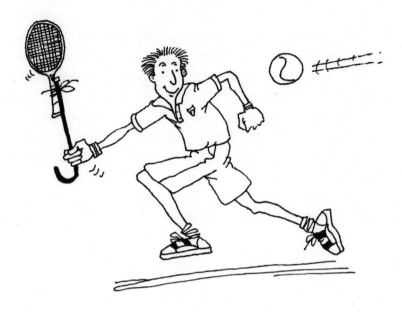

up in other sports too – with rugby, football and hockey all providing ways to participate. Many sports also have five-year age groups such as the Women's Over 45's Cup in hockey or the Wales Over 55 national hockey team. Rugby is a big contact sport, of course, and one definition of a veteran in that sport is 'someone who is too dumb to realise that rugby is a young man's sport'. In the societies in Japan which are long-lived, many men continue with their martial arts, adapted to recognise that one of the effects of growing older is a higher risk of injury and a longer recovery time.

Sports that do not involve body-to-body contact, such as rowing, are of course less risky, but even sports like tennis or golf present challenges. There is a higher risk of muscle and ligament damage in all sports but, as with other problems after the age of 40, the effects of ageing are less significant than the effects of 15 or 20 years of inactivity, of driving and sitting at a desk. It is essential to put effort into training before returning to competitive sport, even if the competition is only with friends. The training needs to focus principally on suppleness and it may be useful to start with yoga or Pilates or tai chi for a few months before going back to the front row of the scrum.

If you do go back to sport, why not move up a league? The aim is to play the sport better than you did at the point at which you gave it up. Obviously you may notice the effects of loss of fitness, at least in the short term, but you can also aim to become more skilful by taking lessons in tennis or whatever you want to play. Your strength and stamina will return in no time.

Getting fitter through dancing

If competitive sport isn't for you, why don't you try dancing? As Angela Rippon emphasised on the BBC programme *How To Stay Young*, dancing is one of the best forms of exercise. Dancing covers all aspects of fitness:

- **Skill** – It is very good for balance and coordination.
- **Suppleness** – Dancing is good for all the joints. Some dances may be better than others, but all have benefits. So whether you enjoy Scottish country or Latin dancing, get moving!
- **Strength** – Every dance requires control and that is provided by core strength. The more you dance, the more this strength is going to increase. Your legs and thighs will also become much stronger.
- **Stamina** – When you're dancing you need lung strength and muscle strength to keep going. The more you dance, the more this is going to improve.

Getting fitter through swimming

Swimming is a great form of exercise and an even better way to get fit. If you can't swim, it's never too late to learn. Swimming builds stamina, strength and fitness and it is one of the few exercises that provides an all-body workout as nearly all of your muscles are used whilst swimming. It is a low-impact activity that is great for muscle workouts because it carries little risk of injury.

As always, your age shouldn't be a barrier – Michael Phelps qualified for his fifth Olympics on the eve of his 31st birthday (and eventually won five gold medals and one silver medal). It's time to ditch the excuses and get in the pool, for there is

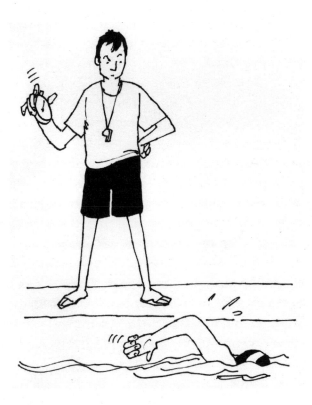

no better time. Use the opportunity of swimming to improve your strength and stamina. It is only a matter of time until you're swimming further and faster.

The first move is to swim a defined distance: 50 or 100 metres, for example, and record your time. This provides the baseline. Now plan your weekly programme. Once or preferably twice a week go to the pool. Over the next three months, challenge yourself to increase the distance you swim, or reduce the time you take to swim a length. Or why not try both?

The next step is to move up a gear but you may need expert help to do so. With the aid of a teacher you can improve your swimming style. The way in which your hand enters the water in the front crawl or the precise movement of the leg kick in the breaststroke can make a big difference to your times. Another breakthrough is to learn a new stroke.

Remember that swimming is not a substitute for your daily strength and suppleness routine; in fact, increasing your daily strength and suppleness training will improve your swimming times.

Getting fitter through cycling

Remember your first bicycle, and the moment when you first managed to ride it without your mum or dad holding the saddle? A new world opened up as a result of your ability to cycle! Next, remember the day you passed the driving test and graduated from the bike to the car, desperate to get off the saddle and behind the wheel. Then, remember the day that you actually got your first car, either buying it or getting it as part of a package for a job that also involved sitting down for seven or eight hours a day. After that it was downhill all the way, putting on weight, feeling tired and increasing your risk of all the 21st-century epidemics.

Now is the time to go back to the bike, the perfect present

for your 40th or 50th birthday, or indeed for your 42nd or 53rd or any other birthday. Or just buy one for yourself and restart cycling, at least five days a week.

Cycling is one of the easiest ways to fit exercise into your daily routine because it's also a form of transport. If you are lucky you can commute on a bike but that is impossible for many people who have to drive a long way to work. Some of them, however, could stick the bike on the back of the car or fold it on the back seat and cycle from the Park and Ride car park or the train station. Again, like swimming, it's a low-impact activity so it's much easier on your joints than, say, running. But it still helps you get into shape. It is an aerobic activity which means your heart, blood vessels and lungs all get a workout. You will breathe deeper and increase your body temperature, which will improve your fitness.

Of course the problem often starts at the office where there is nowhere to store the bike securely and, even rarer, a shower and a place to change. Sooner or later, however, the bosses will learn that encouraging cycling to work is not only good for the workers' health and the environment but also helps people work better.

There is one problem with cycling – it can be too easy. Cycling is a very efficient way of moving and unless you have to cycle up hills you can turn the pedal a few times and then freewheel for a long way. So if you want to cycle to get fit, make sure you are cycling fast enough to feel your pulse rate increase a little and from time to time cycle hard enough to make yourself too breathless to talk.

If you use a stationary cycle in a gym or health club, why not integrate a HIIT workout:

- 5 minutes: Warm-up
- 20 seconds: High intensity; 40 seconds recovery
- 30 seconds: High intensity; 30 seconds recovery
- 20 seconds: High intensity; 40 seconds recovery

Getting fitter through pilates, yoga, tai chi, kung fu and the alexander technique

There are other activities that you can do to increase your strength, stamina and suppleness.

These activities not only develop your strength and fitness, but they also:

- Encourage you to clear your mind and focus on your body, not on your next meal or your last argument
- Involve all the muscles and joints of the body: the upper and lower limbs, core muscles of the abdomen and back, the spine and neck
- Increase and improve strength, suppleness and skill: the skill of balance, for example
- Help you learn exercises that you can use on your own, either in a half-hour session, or built into your ten-minute daily schedule, or done in two minutes before a stressful meeting or after an hour sitting at a keyboard

Of course there are differences between them, differences felt very strongly by those who are committed to one particular discipline, but from your point of view just choose any one of the four that a friend is doing or that you hear has a good teacher. There is a cost, but that cost is much less if you join a class, or ask a teacher to come for even one session to a club or something you belong to. Also, why not suggest to your boss or manager that even one session would pay for itself with the added energy that you and your colleagues would have, not only that day but also in the days and weeks that follow.

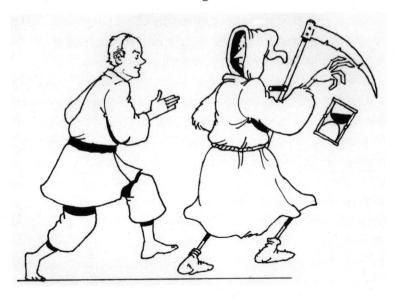

Getting fitter in a gym

Some people love them, some people hate them, but gyms and fitness clubs are health services. Start by looking at your local council website and type in the word fitness. Councils have had 'leisure centres' for decades but, partly because the word leisure conjures up a picture of lying back on a sofa with a pina colada, the emphasis is changing to sports and fitness and, of course, local authorities have swimming pools too. Increasingly, councils are developing fitness trails in their parks and these trails often have equipment and advice at key points in the circuit.

If you can afford it, joining a gym is a motivating experience and the novelty of the equipment is another stimulus. Good old-fashioned weights – dumb-bells and barbells – are making a big comeback but you need advice from a trainer before you start pumping iron because technique is of great importance. Weights are increasingly popular with women, as is boxing, reflecting the fact that people don't just want to take exercise to lose weight but to gain muscle. Why not aim to lift half your weight within six months?

If you join a gym you will meet the trainers who run classes but you may want to find a trainer yourself, and you don't need to be a gym member to do this. In times past, training was the activity you did to prepare for sport and trainers were focused on boxers or football teams. Over the years the world has changed and trainers are now probably helping more office workers rather than football players. The term personal trainer was introduced in the USA, a personal trainer being someone who would help top executives and millionaires become fitter and look better, especially the latter.

Over the years, however, trainers evolved as fitness clubs, leisure centres and gyms attracted people who were not millionaires but who realised the dangers of their sedentary lifestyle and the benefits of exercise. Some people can just turn up at a gym and do their stuff but many people prefer to join a spinning club or step class or use some of the elaborate equipment and they need the help of a trainer; one-to-one training is not always necessary, although nice if you can afford it, and trainers are trained not only to coach and encourage but to make classes inclusive and fun.

Getting fitter with a personal trainer

You have taken the first step and made the decision to get in better shape. That is fantastic, but now what? If at all possible, getting a personal trainer is the best plan: someone who is trained to help you achieve your goals, whatever they may be, and also to help motivate and push you more than you probably would on your own. But how do you choose the right PT for you? There are a lot of them out there and many can be quite pushy about trying to get new clients (you can't blame them, really, since they are usually self-employed).

There are many factors to take into consideration:

- What kind of vibe do you want your sessions to have; do you want it to be all business or would you prefer someone a bit more relaxed and chatty? It's important to get on with your PT.
- What kind of motivational techniques work best for you? Do you want someone to be shouting at you (some people love this!) or do you want lots of gentle positive reinforcement. If you know, then tell your trainer.
- What are your training goals? All trainers will have slightly different ways of doing things and most will have areas they specialise in (e.g. strength training, long-distance running, boxing) so it's important to find someone who fits in with what you are aiming for.
- Ask how they train themselves, as that will give a good indication as to their areas of expertise. Also, if you have aims in line with how they like to train themselves the sessions are likely to be more enjoyable because the PT is sharing their passion.
- Ask questions and don't be afraid to tell them if there is anything you particularly love or hate while exercising. There will be some things you like, even if you don't know what yet! And if this is the case, it's the PT's job to figure out, with you, what those things are.
- Remember that you are paying them to help you achieve your goals: they have to listen to you. There is no point in them setting you a programme full of things you detest because you will not do them on your own. For your lifestyle change to be long term, you will need to be able to do it on your own unless

you are lucky enough to see a PT several times a week. Be honest and realistic with your trainer when it comes to planning your programme. It's better to commit to working out once a week between sessions and doing so, maybe more often, than saying you'll work out three times and not managing it. Having this information will help them devise the best programme for you.

- Decide how much nutritional advice you want. Some PTs are qualified to give an eating plan and some won't have done the appropriate courses for that. You may or may not want or need help about your food but it's worth looking at it a little bit at least as it will make a difference to how you respond to your new exercise plan and how you feel.

- Ask them about their qualifications and experience. They should at a minimum have a Level 3 Personal Training qualification. On top of this they will most likely have done shorter courses in things like nutrition or certain types of exercise, for example strength and conditioning, kettle-bells, MMA (mixed martial arts) training or endurance training.

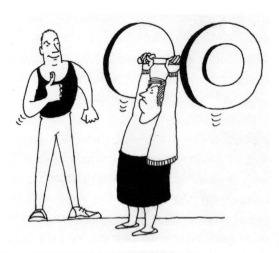

Once you have chosen your PT and started training with them there are some things to keep in mind:

- There is a direct relationship between the effort you put in and the results you will see and feel.
- Be honest (with your trainer and also yourself). If you've slacked off then admit it and recommit. If you know the reason you haven't been following the programme they have set for you then talk to them about it and find a solution.
- Don't quit. It will be hard at first but it will be worth it if you stick with it.
- Be realistic. There is a direct correlation between the amount of time and effort you put in to the results you will see and feel.

Increasingly the NHS and others are recognising the benefits of training. So fitness trainers are now becoming one step on the care pathway for people with back pain and they will be included in many more pathways for long-term health problems in the years to come.

Getting fit with technology

Remember the pedometer? It was a technological device that was revolutionary in helping people measure how much walking they were doing, and motivating them to walk more.

It is now redundant because of the development of more sophisticated technology, epitomised by the Fitbit and a wide range of what is now called 'wearable technology', ranging from simpler and less expensive wristbands to devices with many more functions. Fitbit itself is now available in many different forms, with additional functions at increased cost, and there are competitors at every level (the Microsoft Band, for example).

Phones are also changing. First they were mobile and now they are smart. Most phones now have apps and there are some fantastic ones available to download. Walkmeter and Runmeter, for example, can be used to measure how much you walk or run. I have already talked about the Couch to 5K app from the One You compaign; it is a great app which is designed to get you off the couch and running in just nine weeks.

Smart watches are another new trend, with the iWatch leading the way. These watches can not only measure how much exercise you are taking, but they can even remind you to stand up regularly if you are in a desk job.

One of the benefits of technology is to provide you with feedback and motivation. Another benefit is that it can help you enjoy getting fit with other people (even though you never see them because they are in other parts of the country or even in other countries). But you don't need to spend vast amounts of money for special technology to get fit – all you need is yourself and the right attitude. Websites such as MyFitnessPal allow you to share information about food and exercise for support and competition.

Getting fitter with a dog

Is there a single gene for loving of dogs and cats? People are either 'dog people' or 'cat people', or they love both, or they dislike both intensely. It is a bit like blood group: people are either A or B, or A B if they have both genes, or O if they have neither. Surprisingly, perhaps, the world's geneticists do not seem to be focused on this intriguing issue. What researchers are doing, however, is studying the effects of pet ownership on health. The prestigious Harvard Medical School has even published a Special Health Report with the title 'Get Healthy, Get a Dog'.

There are a few adverse results of pet ownership, of which

allergy and financial pressures are the most common, but the overall effect is positive, provided of course that you are a dog person or a cat person, although there are reports of people who were firmly in the anti-pet brigade being won over by the stray puppy from the rescue shelter or a kitten. The positive effects are significant. For cats they are primarily on mental well-being but dogs improve both mental and physical health, particularly helping with weight control. A dog is an excellent antidote to the sedentary life, particularly beneficial for home-workers because no matter how strongly that email is calling out for reply, a dog with its ball in its mouth is an even stronger call to action. Even if you don't or can't own a dog there may be one nearby whose owner is no longer able to take it for the exercise it needs and would welcome a walker's help.

Birthday and christmas present list

Make it clear that although it is the thought that counts, a huge box of chocolates would not be welcome as a present. (It may be, of course, that the giver wants you to eat your way to an early grave!) To make it easier for your nearest and dearest, here are some ideas for presents, although you can get fitter without spending a penny. Here are some gifts for fitness:

1. A resistance band – stretchy rubber for upper body exercise
2. Weights – either a pair of little dumb-bells of 3 or 5kg, or kettle-bells
3. A Fitbit or similar exercise tracker such as the more expensive but cool Microsoft Band to wear proudly round your wrist, although you can get many of the features of these exercise trackers on your mobile phone using apps like the Walkmeter

4. Swimming lessons or lessons for other sports. Even if you already swim, lessons help you to swim better and faster
5. A lesson or two or a course of yoga, tai chi, Pilates or the Alexander technique to learn exercises you can build into your daily routine

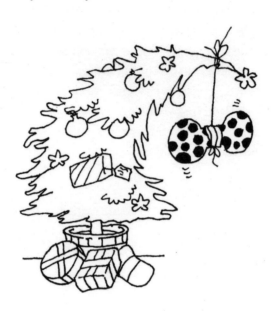

Part Four

Healthy Eating

Resources on eating well	What's in it for you
Health Check	At the Health Check you will have your height and weight measured so that your BMI can be calculated. If your BMI is high you will be offered a test for type 2 diabetes
One You	The How Are You quiz asks, how often you snack, how many helpings of fruit and vegetables you eat and what your food choices are
Your annual review if you have a long-term condition like type 2 diabetes or high blood pressure	Healthier eating should be included in your annual review but the time is often fully taken up with reviewing your drugs so if you are not asked about eating and food use the How Are You quiz
NHS Choices	There is a lot of good information, for example: • The 12-week weight loss guide • Eight tips for healthy eating • What is a Mediterranean diet?
High-quality apps	Try the Sugar Smart app and the One You Easy Meals app

When the subject of smoking comes up in a Health Check or the How Are You quiz everyone is clear about the right answer. With exercise it is also pretty clear, we should almost all be doing more, but with diet, what are the right answers?

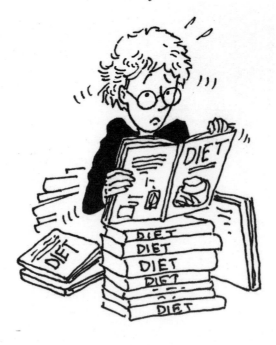

Dieticians, academics and physicians all disagree. But there is a core knowledge that everyone agrees on and that it what we will look at in this section.

Diet, then, is a really, really, confusing topic. Just think how many people are writing books, appearing on TV, Instagramming, tweeting and blogging on food, diet and health. There are hundreds of diets all making claims that sound very convincing. Then there are celebrities who make promises about their methods, all without what would be called evidence in the medical world.

How well are you eating?

The evidence base about exercise is much stronger than the evidence base about diet. Experts all differ on what you should eat more of but actually they are very consistent on

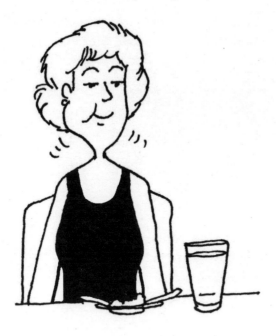

what you should eat less of and the best way to describe it is to use a phrase popular in the USA: Eat Less Crap.

There is no doubt that Americans eat a lot of crap, as the sign 'Deep-Fried Dough' at every baseball stadium testifies, but Britain is close behind in the race to become the most obese nation on earth.

It is, however, not just obesity that is the problem. There is little doubt that what we eat has an influence on the risk of developing many common diseases. The problem is that experts disagree and change their minds frequently and new experts emerge every month with their miracle diets.

Eating 'crap' increases the risk of developing disease in later life and makes you feel less well now, so let's start with our crap detector:

How often do you consume these things?	Score 3 for most days of the week, 2 for some days a week and 1 for never
Biscuits	
Sweets	
Salty packaged snacks	
Sweet packaged snacks	
Cans of sugar-rich soft drinks	

- If you scored 6, well done.
- If you scored under 12, there is still scope for eating better and feeling better.
- If you scored more than 12 but less than 18, you need to take action.

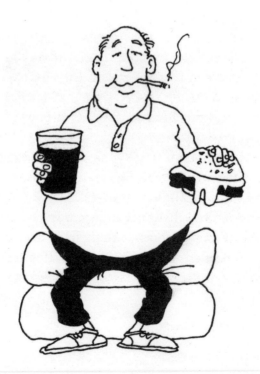

- If you scored 18, you really need to get a grip because you are consuming way too much salt and sugar.

The salt cellar and the sugar bowl are not the principal culprits, however, on which we can blame our modern diet and its consequences, namely:

- obesity
- type 2 diabetes
- heart disease
- stroke
- high blood pressure
- some cancers, notably breast and colorectal

With salt and sugar the message is simple: eat less. In midlife especially, you need to consume less of both. The best way to do this is not to throw away your salt cellar and sugar bowl, although you should put them out of sight and not on the table for every meal. The big source of salt and sugar is in ready-made food and therefore you need to pay more attention to the snacks or ready-made meals you buy, probably without thinking when you are in a rush. You can use the new Sugar Smart app from Public Health England to check just how much sugar is in the package or bottle on the shelf.

Less salt, less sugar. This is the easy part of the story. The remainder is a little more complicated. But it is worthwhile to try to understand the issues and the reasons for the disagreements because there are two good reasons to change your diet, either to lose weight or to reduce the risk of disease, and fortunately the changes are virtually the same for both.

How is your weight?

Firstly, decide if you need to lose weight. Here are three simple questions. If you answer 'yes' to one or more, you need to get a grip, otherwise you will be 5kg heavier at the age of 60, and 10kg more at 70.

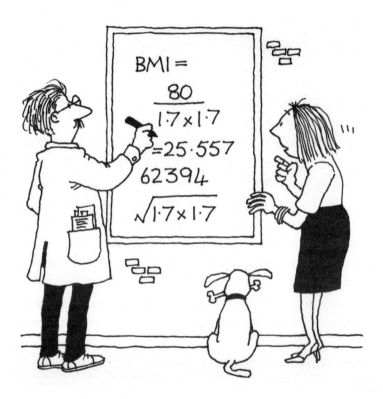

One way to identify how healthy you are is to calculate your BMI. Almost everyone nowadays knows about the body mass index even if they don't know their own BMI. The BMI has been around since the 1830s, when the formula on which it is based was developed by Lambert Adolphe Jacques Quetelet (1796–1874), a Belgian astronomer, mathematician and statistician. The formula is that your BMI equals your weight in kilograms divided by your height in metres, multiplied by itself.

$$BMI = \frac{\text{Weight in kilograms}}{\text{Height in metres x Height in metres}}$$

(For example, for a man weighing 80kg and 1.7m)

$$BMI = \frac{80}{1.7 \text{ X } 1.7} = 25.5$$

The term body mass index was coined in 1972 by an epidemiologist (a scientist who studies the health of populations) called Ancel Keys and it is widely used in spite of the fact that it is less relevant in people who are black or Asian, and there are calls for it to be changed. Nick Trefethen, a very distinguished professor of mathematics at Oxford, has argued that instead of your height being multiplied by itself, which mathematicians call being squared or raised to the power of two, it should be raised to the power of 2.5. The advantages and disadvantages of doing this are difficult for non-mathematicians to understand so the BMI in some form will probably remain a key marker of your risk for years to come.

The BMI does not suit everyone. For people who are fit and have a lot of muscle, it can be frustrating to be told that their BMI indicates that they are overweight or even obese. The BMI is designed for the average human being and people who have above average muscle mass and have put on muscle are better using the BFP (body fat percentage). Look online to find the formula.

Now, let's have a look at your health.

	Yes or no
Are you heavier than you were at 30?	
Are you now buying trousers with a bigger waist or a bigger dress size than at 20?	
When you look in a mirror naked, do you think you would look better with less weight?	

The increase in weight that takes place as many people grow older is almost always due not only to an increased intake of food or alcohol, but also to decreased energy expenditure as a consequence of inactivity. Your genes play a part in your

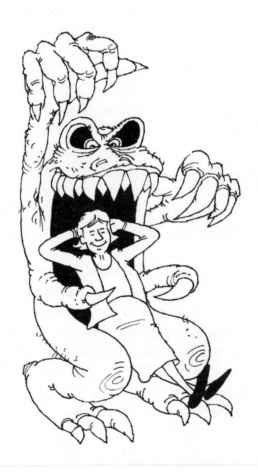

struggle against gaining weight but it is best to think of obesity as a 21st-century epidemic caused by the world in which we live and then to develop techniques to adapt to and cope with this dangerous environment.

Weight gain is therefore the other side of the coin to loss of fitness, and the solution is the same – increase energy expenditure and decrease energy intake.

This will not result in rapid weight loss, but the strategy to improve your stamina by walking for 30 minutes extra for five days a week and getting breathless twice a week will both help you lose weight and prevent you regaining the weight you have lost by reducing your intake of energy. Taking exercise for 30 minutes is of benefit, but increasing attention is now focused on the other 15 or more hours of waking time. James Levine, a British doctor working at the Mayo Clinic Obesity Solutions Initiative, points out in a book called *Get Up!*, wonderfully subtitled 'Why your chair is killing you and what you can do about it', that if we define exercise as exertion for the sake of developing fitness then many people do not take exercise, and for many of those who do, the amount of energy expended (about 200 calories in a session) is much less than they expend in the rest of the 24 hours (about 2,000 calories). He calls the energy used in activities other than exercise NEAT, for non-exercise activity thermogenesis, the word thermogenesis meaning energy burning. He writes that his research suggests that some people have a NEAT switch, which switches on and makes them get up and move about if they consume more calories than they need, so that they sit less than people who do not have this switch, who sit and get fat. So, if you are the sort of person who puts on weight easily then it might be that you do not have a NEAT switch; to control your weight you have to be aware of the need to stand, for example to stand every hour for at least five minutes and to do a lot of little stand-ups, for example to stand up ten times, at least in every ad break.

If you put too much petrol into your car the surplus spurts back onto your hands and shoes, but your body does not have an energy tank which will only hold so much like your car's petrol tank. If you take in more energy than you need the surplus is converted to fat, and for a very good reason. That is, it is only in the last few centuries that food supply in winter has been secure. In hard times it was an advantage to lay down fat. People whose genetic code was such that they deposited fat when there was a surplus of food in summer months were more likely to survive, and to breed the following summer. So there are genetic factors which influence how efficient we are at laying down fat, but nonetheless, some people have to be more careful about their energy balance than others. Everyone can put on weight if they consume more energy than they need, and everyone can lose weight if they change their energy balance.

To reduce your energy intake you need to reduce your intake of foods that are high in energy and low in volume, the volume being important because if your stomach is not filled you will feel hungry soon afterwards. So eat less of – or, better, stop eating completely – the stuff listed in the table near the beginning of this chapter. It is also important to remember that alcohol is calorie-rich, so cutting back on alcohol makes a contribution to reducing your energy intake.

How much alcohol should we drink?

People in their midlife are usually the generation who started using drugs other than, or in addition to, alcohol seriously when in their twenties and some people continue to do so, but alcohol is a greater health problem than other drugs in midlife. The problem comes from both dependence and its impact on physical health, particularly liver disease and weight gain. As with other risk factors there is no limit above which you are 'at risk' and below which you are 'safe', but neither is it helpful simply to advise people to 'drink less' or 'drink carefully', so here are the guidelines from the Department of Health:

- Don't drink more than 14 units a week, i.e.
  - 6 pints of beer or
  - 6 glasses of wine or
  - 14 small shots of spirit.
- Don't drink this amount all on one day.
- Do have two or more alcohol-free days every week.

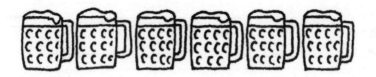

Stopping alcohol for a month is also a good move because it is rich in calories. The Dry January campaign www.dryjanuary.org.uk is one way to do this, but you could also do Dry June or Dry November! For many people cutting back on alcohol in midlife makes good sense in any case because you are not so resilient, and the effects of alcohol are more powerful.

Resources on avoiding alcohol problems	What's in it for you
Health Check	The Health Check uses a checklist called AUDIT
One You	The How Are You quiz asks how many days of the week you drink alcohol and on those days how many units of alcohol you put away

(continued)

Resources on avoiding alcohol problems	What's in it for you
Your annual review if you have a long-term condition like type 2 diabetes or high blood pressure	This is unlikely to be raised except for people having a review because they have liver disease so you will need to rely on NHS Choices, which has good resources for you to consult
NHS Choices	NHS Choices has a very wide range of different resources and information, including: • Calories in alcohol • Binge drinking • Tips on cutting down • Caring for an alcoholic Just type 'alcohol' into the NHS Choices search box
High-quality apps	Try the One You Drinks Tracker

Many people find it helpful to start their weight loss plan with a fixed period of time. NHS Choices has a 12-week plan to help you bring about this transformation, and some people find what they call '5 plus 2' helpful – that is, 2 days a week fasting.

One means of support in this effort is to keep reminding yourself that the same changes that will help you lose weight will also reduce the risk of you developing many of the common diseases that cause early disability and death.

Eat better, look younger: go mediterranean

Part of the reason why there is much less emphasis on what we eat as a cause of death and disability than on smoking is that the experts are in disarray. The plethora of faddy diets and new diets, good fat/bad fat arguments, and cooking and baking programmes on television are evidence of the confusion that exists. However, it does appear that some agreement is developing on what we should eat and how we should eat it.

One reason for the confusion is that what people eat varies dramatically and it is almost impossible to organise research to answer the big questions. The research therefore rarely produces clear-cut results and the people who study diet and health have to use their judgement when they interpret the results of their research. I have therefore used my judgement in weighing up the claims of different researchers.

Every month new miracle diets appear and they usually focus on some particular aspect of the diet – red meat or cheese or tofu or fish – that is recommended as one thing you need to eat more, or less, of. However, almost all of these miracle diets include the principles of what is called the Mediterranean diet: the diet eaten in Italy, France, Greece, Spain and other countries on the northern shores of the Mediterranean can be recommended. This diet has been associated with good health, including a healthier heart. A 2013 study found that people following the Mediterranean diet had a 30 per cent lower risk of heart disease and stroke. The diet is very similar to the Eatwell Guide set out by the UK government. It is based on vegetables, fruits, nuts, beans, cereal grains, olive oil and fish.

NHS Choices has a very clear description of the key elements of the Mediterranean diet and the following foods can be eaten in abundance:

- Fruit and vegetables – not just five a day but seven a day if you wish. There is one new bit of advice that is emerging: 'eat purple'. Purple foods are associated with a longer life because they contain polyphenols,

so eat more red cabbage, blackcurrants and
blueberries

- Nuts, peas and beans – for their low-fat protein
- Brown bread, brown rice and other wholemeal food
  and grains – for their fibre
- Pulses and lentils – for the chemical called inulin
- Olive oil – for the unsaturated fats

Go for it, eat as much as you want from the list above. However, whilst it is important to incorporate as many of these
foods as possible in your everyday diet, you don't need to do
so at every meal. It might be easier to try and get the balance
right over a longer period of time – such as a week, a month,
or even a year!

The traditional description of the Mediterranean diet
emphasises the daily glass of red wine but this does not
appear to be essential and has probably been promoted by
someone looking to justify their daily tipple. My advice is to
have at least two alcohol-free days a week, even if you are on
the Mediterranean diet.

The Benefits Of Red Wine

Red wine's reputation is based not only on its Mediterranean
connection. It is also given credit for what has been called the
French paradox, namely the fact that French people, even in
the windy north of France, far from the Mediterranean,
apparently consume large quantities of Brie and Camembert
but have a lower rate of heart disease than in the UK. So what
is the effect of red wine?

First the good news: provided you do not exceed the weekly
limit of 14 units of alcohol, less than five large glasses of wine,
red wine has some beneficial effects on heart health. The effect
comes not from the alcohol but from chemicals called

(continued)

polyphenols. These are present in much higher concentrations in red wine than in white wine because the grape skins are removed in the making of white wine. Differences in fermenting techniques result in some reds having higher polyphenol concentrations than others and it seems that polyphenols are beneficial because they cause blood vessels to dilate. Polyphenols are antioxidants which protect cells from harmful chemicals and the polyphenol that is receiving a lot of attention, certainly in websites such as www.winefrog.com, is called resveratrol.

That's the good news. The not-so-good news, certainly for people hoping to justify the consumption of red wine on health grounds, is that many other foodstuffs contain polyphenols, so instead of a glass of wine the same effect could be obtained by eating a bowl of cranberries or a small handful of walnuts or drinking a nice strong cup of tea.

Eating less

Number one on the 'eat less' list is anything that is offered in a shiny package near or on the way to the till. When it comes to the more basic ingredients, almost everyone recommends less white flour and more wholemeal for the fibre.

For fat, the story is more complicated but getting simpler. The scientific evidence is confusing but there are a few general principles about fat which most (but not all) experts agree on, and which are worth basing your shopping, cooking and eating on.

- Reduce saturated fats, which are principally animal fats, found in red meat, butter and cream; red meat can be replaced by what is called white meat – chicken (or other poultry) and oily fish.

- Increase unsaturated fats from plants, notably olive oil or oil from nuts. Not all vegetable oil is recommended – corn oil, for example, is not.
- Try to eat oily fish – salmon, mackerel or tuna, fresh not tinned – at least twice a week.
- Avoid hydrogenated fat or 'trans fat' – it's always on the label.

There is also a very good, long list of things you can and should eat more of, not just to stave off hunger but because they contain valuable elements.

There have been studies of people who live in populations in which health in advanced old age is common, such as Okinawa, Sardinia and Icaria, which are called 'Blue Zones'. A Blue Zone is a geographic or demographic area of the world where people live longer, happier and healthier lives.

All the Blue Zones have distinctive diets, but the Mediterranean diet is probably more relevant and acceptable to Britain than the diet of Okinawa. It may be, of course, that the diet in the Blue Zones is not actually affecting the ageing process but simply allowing people to live the full lifespan of 90 or 100 years which, for many of us, is cut short by preventable disease, because many of these diseases are caused by the diet that we eat. It is also important to emphasise that the people in the Blue Zones don't just eat differently, they have a number of distinctive features. Perhaps the key message from Sardinia is, as I have emphasised, 'Don't worry about ageing, just keep fit, have the right attitude and eat like us.'

How to eat

If you have a definitive lunch hour with a canteen nearby offering bowls of salad, it is easier to eat well and take a ten-minute walk than if you are driving a taxi or a lorry, or working in an office or factory far from home with no canteen or kitchen. Time pressures, the physical surroundings, and the general hassle and stress of work make it difficult to eat well at midday. But it is possible to eat well at home and to take some of the techniques and tips listed below to work.

In Okinawa, the Japanese island that is one of the Blue Zones, people repeat a slogan before they start to eat – *hara hachi bu* – which reminds them that they are not going to eat till they are at bursting point. Instead, they will stop eating when they are quite full but not completely full.

Here are some things you can do to stop you overeating:

- Don't read or watch television when eating, otherwise you can finish up with an empty plate but no memory of having eaten anything.
- Eat slowly, putting your knife and fork down between every mouthful.
- Use smaller plates.

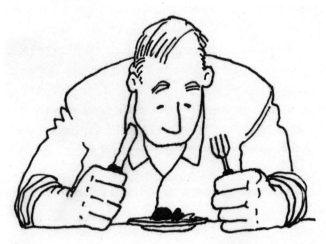

- Put the foods you should avoid – biscuits and cakes, sugar bowls and salt cellars – out of sight.
- Sit down to eat, even if you are very rushed.
- Concentrate for a minute before you start eating.

People in their forties and fifties face one additional risk factor for obesity – children. 'Dad's bod' is a newly-discovered condition which is appropriately named, with some researchers showing that weight increases when the family arrives. One possible reason is that Dad often clears the unfinished food on children's plates! So to prevent Dad's (and Mum's) bod, put less on their plates in the first place, and that will have the additional benefit of contributing to the prevention of another modern epidemic – childhood obesity.

Support for healthy eating

The two principal supports that the health service can offer to people who want to lose weight are appetite suppressants and surgery to shrink the size of the stomach. Neither option is relevant for most people. The drugs have adverse side effects and are of limited efficacy, and the surgery is suitable only for a very few people. However, the world-famous Harvard Medical School's report 'Healthy Solutions to Lose Weight and Keep It Off' emphasises that research demonstrates plenty of things you can do. The report highlights the need to see this as a change in the way you lead your life and cope with the stressful environment in which you live, not just a one-off campaign, and offers '10 habits to help you lose weight'. Here are their tips and my advice on how to put them into practice.

Tips from Harvard Medical School report	My advice
Start self-monitoring	Weigh yourself at the same time every week
Create a behaviour chain	Start getting fitter at the same time as you start losing weight

(*continued*)

Tips from Harvard Medical School report	My advice
Get a support network	Join a group like Slimming World or Weight Watchers or the Hairy Bikers' Diet Club or start a group with friends or in the office
Energise your exercise	See Part Three
Make sure you're getting enough sleep	See Part Two
Eat breakfast slowly and mindfully every day	Don't eat while watching TV; put your knife and fork down after every mouthful
Monitor and modify your screen time	Do less sitting; if you have to spend time at the computer, sit less and stand more
Shop smarter	Use the Sugar Smart app
Reward yourself with (non-food) pleasures	Say no more!

Of these ten tips, 'Get a support network' is the most important. There are now apps to let you join a virtual community, which is great for those who have a busy, frantic lifestyle. For many people, men in particular, the virtual community offers the advantage of belonging but at the same time protecting your privacy and not having to reveal your weight or your emotions.

Face-to-face communication, however, is still one of the best ways to get support. The community can be informal, just you and your family, for example, or formal. Two great examples are Weight Watchers and Slimming World.

Weight Watchers and Slimming World are very well-known organisations but their brand, namely how they are perceived by people who are not overweight, is not well understood. To people who are not members it is all too easy to assume that Weight Watchers and Slimming World will focus on diet and exercise, but this is not the case. The image of these organisations held by many people who have never joined is not very positive. The image is of a hall filled with women weighing one another, applauding those who have lost weight and encouraging in various ways, not all of them sympathetic, those who have not lost weight.

This is not a true picture of how Weight Watchers and Slimming World work. Firstly, many people are now online members and the emails they receive when they sign up are very encouraging. Here are some samples of the opening lines. There is not a mention of calories or dieting; instead the Weight Watchers website says 'We know how tempting it is to measure women's success by just the number on the scale but that's only part of it.' 'Success is not just about what you lose – it's about everything you gain: it's about having a healthier and happier life.'

You are then encouraged to 'set aside time for yourself' and make an action plan, not to eat more vegetables but to schedule 'some me-time: anything that falls under the "three R's" counts – relaxation, recreation and restoration'. Then it moves on to give practical advice on how to do the three R's, for example:

- If you have 4 minutes – take a deep breath – close your eyes, inhale for five counts. Rest and repeat.
- If you have 10 minutes . . . start a mini journal – even if it's one sentence a day to reflect on something positive or funny.
- If you have 15 minutes or more . . . just unplug – turn off the mobile, the iPad and the TV. Digital detoxes are all the rage and you will feel better afterwards.

Finally, and still no mention of calories, the initial email gives you the following tips:

- Find more me time every day
- Get – and stay – happy
- Define your success, check out our basic plan on goal setting: where do you want to be?

As I have tried to do in this book, Weight Watchers encourages you to think about yourself and your environment and its pressures before giving advice or information.

The Slimming World approach is very similar; here is what their website says:

> To change the habits that have formed over years — sometimes decades — slimmers need in-depth support and encouragement, and that's so much more than praise on a good week and commiseration for a bad week. . . . At the heart of our friendly groups is a powerfully motivating session we call IMAGE Therapy. IMAGE stands for Individual Motivation And Group Experience. It's the part of the group where everyone benefits from the experiences of their fellow members – to help change habits, share healthy swaps, make decisions about the week ahead, to uncover any old habits that might be slowing your weight loss and develop strategies to overcome them.

Slimming World also recognises that not everyone will want or be able to join a group and offers online membership with a number of online resources, such as:

- Look to the future with **Visualisation** – a relaxing audio-feature to help you to achieve and, more importantly, maintain your new slim shape.
- The **SAS log** is an incredibly powerful tool that will help you discover where you might be subconsciously sabotaging your weight loss and aim to make subtle changes each day until self-sabotage is a thing of the past.

- Make a **For & Against** list – and tap into the deeper reasons which have shaped how you behave today and which may make you resist being slim.

There is no direct comparison of these two services and the local groups will vary depending on the leadership. Ask around and choose a group or go online and select which appeals more. Also, the image of these organisations is of gatherings of women and while it is true that most people who go to meetings are women, men are welcome. However, men may prefer the online membership, or they may prefer to join a new group online set up by two male midlifers – the Big Hairy Bikers' Diet Club.

Don't dig your grave with your teeth

Eating a healthy, balanced diet is an important part of maintaining good health. Not only will changing the way you eat make you feel better, it will also make your skin look younger and help you feel more energetic. By eating a wide variety of foods, in the right proportions, you will stay healthy and live longer. However, it is not only your diet that needs to change. There are also other aspects of your life that can be altered.

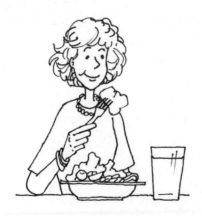

Part Five

Everyday Health

When bookies are setting the odds for a race, they are trying to estimate the odds on a horse winning. To do this, they have to gather information from a number of sources and from their own knowledge. They don't have time to go and look at the horses walking round the ring because by that time they are busy collecting bets. They also take into account the environment – the 'going', as they call it.

If you have health insurance, the insurance company does the same thing as the bookie; they try to estimate your risk of dying early and charge you accordingly. The NHS and the public health service take a different approach. They want to

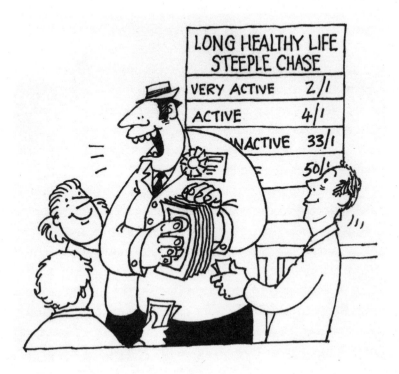

help you understand and reduce your risk of disease and disability. Sometimes the task is relatively straightforward, and where a single risk factor such as your age is the main risk and there is a proven test available, it is possible to screen for particular diseases.

We keep talking about health care as though that is what other people do for you, but health care is what you do for yourself; health services are what the professionals provide. The best person to look after your body regularly is yourself and here is what you can do to keep your body in good trim.

Information about health and risks to health is often given in round numbers such as 'Men should not drink more than 14 units of alcohol a week' or 'Eat 5 portions of fruit or vegetables every day'. These round numbers should not lead you to believe that they are absolute. No, it is not as simple as that. Instead, it is all a matter of risk and determining exactly what that particular risk has on your health and well-being. Sir David Spiegelhalter describes this very clearly in his website www.understandinguncertainty.org.

The word risk is a difficult term and the experts have a number of definitions but the one common to all is that it is a probability that some event will happen. Some experts restrict it to adverse events, whilst some use the word for both good and bad events. (However, throughout this book 'risk' is used only to refer to bad events whilst the word 'chance' relates to good events.)

It is also important to understand that your perception of risk is affected by the way in which the risk is described. It is now clear that people, both patients and doctors, make different decisions depending on how the information is presented. If information is presented in relative terms, for example that there is a 10 per cent reduction in risk, the person is much more likely to accept the offer of treatment than if absolute numbers are used, for example by stating that 'For every 1,000 women who take drug X for 10 years (instead of a placebo), there will be 1 less breast cancer death.' This is from a book called *Know Your Chances* by Steve Woloshin, Lisa Schwartz and Gilbert Welch. Furthermore, many doctors do not understand how to communicate risks without bias, as Gerd Gigerenzer, who has studied risk communication, says in his book *Reckoning with Risk: Learning to Live with Uncertainty*: 'Many physicians still have difficulties drawing diagnostic inferences from statistics.'

This all becomes very important when you start thinking about ways in which you can reduce your risk of coming to a bad end, and you need to be clear about the benefits offered when considering either primary prevention, stopping disease from starting in the first place, or screening, identifying it early.

Now, let's have a look at the areas of your health in which you can identify risk and start to make the changes that will affect your health and well-being.

Your heart and blood vessels

In the last 20 years, there has been a dramatic fall in deaths from heart disease. This is in part due to better treatment, but it is also due to the preventive measures that people are taking. The advice in the previous chapters about diet and fitness will reduce your risk of developing and dying from disease of the heart and blood vessels – the nation's number-one killer. In addition, all the steps you take to reduce your risk of heart disease will also help your heart to function better here and now.

During your NHS Health Check, if you are identified as being at high risk of heart disease or stroke then you will be offered treatment for the factors that increase risk, notably:

- high blood pressure
- high blood sugar, also known as type 2 diabetes

- high levels of cholesterol
- smoking

However, unless the levels, and therefore the risks, are extremely high you could ask your doctor, 'What additional risk would I run if I postponed starting the drug treatment for a year and sorted out my diet, my weight and my fitness?' You will be surprised by the answers. It is always best to alter your diet and fitness before participating in drug treatment. Not only will you feel better, but also your health and well-being will infinitely improve. There is one special case. If your father, or one or more other relatives, died of a heart attack before the age of 50 you might have a rare genetic disorder called familial hypercholesterolaemia and you should ask for a genetic test.

Everything you do to lower your risk of heart disease acts by keeping the arteries that supply the heart itself with oxygen healthy; the bonus is that all the arteries of your body will also stay healthy longer and that includes the arteries to the brain.

Your brain

The one disease that most people fear even more than cancer is dementia, but for the first time in 2015 scientific research found evidence that the risk of dementia was decreasing.

Alzheimer's disease, the commonest type of dementia, is not preventable, although there are some hopeful signs that an effective treatment will be found. However, many people develop dementia because the blood vessels to the brain become narrowed by the same disease process that can cause a heart attack – atherosclerosis. When this disease affects the arteries of the brain it can cause either a stroke, if a big artery is blocked, or dementia, if lots of small arteries are progressively narrowed and blocked.

By reducing the risk factors for heart disease you can therefore also reduce the risk of dementia, which is very good news, and this does not simply mean taking pills for high blood pressure or type 2 diabetes. What is becoming apparent is that activity has a beneficial effect on the brain, not just mental activity but physical activity – any physical activity, but the more vigorous the better! Physical activity keeps the blood vessels to the brain healthy by preventing inflammation and this keeps the brain itself healthy. So the evidence is clear. NICE, the National Institute for Health and Care Excellence, which reviews all the scientific evidence and advises the NHS on what works and what doesn't, is emphatic that it is possible to 'delay or prevent the onset of dementia, disability and frailty' by taking action in midlife.

Your lungs

Getting fitter not only increases your mental well-being, but will also help you feel less breathless. This is because training increases the ability of the muscles to suck oxygen from the blood that is passing through them rather than from a direct action of the lungs themselves. The other big issue is now air pollution, particularly from diesel engines, which produce nitrogen dioxide (NO_2), and what is needed is to ban these engines from cities. There are some steps you can take if you cannot avoid city-centre life and air, for example:

- Monitor air pollution using an app on your phone and try to avoid smog spots, if you can, on days when levels are particularly high.
- Avoid busy streets with tall buildings on either side.
- Walk on the inside of the pavement, not the kerb.
- Keep car windows shut and don't bring outside air into the car from busy streets.

Eating fresh fruit, vegetables, and whole grains may protect against harmful effects of free radicals, but equally important is to join a campaign for cleaner air in cities or become a councillor in your city and work for a better environment.

Some of the questions in the Health Check interview or the How Are You quiz are difficult to answer accurately – 'How much exercise do you take?', for example. However, there is one question that is easy because there is only one answer – yes or no: 'Do you smoke?'

If the answer is 'yes' the advice is simple – quit smoking. Even if you have tried before – once, twice or even 20 times – please try again. This is important. Support can be found within your family and friends, but there is also a lot of help available online. The best place to start online is the NHS Choices page on quitting smoking. Let's look briefly at the top ten benefits:

1. You will breathe easier – By quitting smoking your lung capacity improves by 10 per cent in the first 9 months and you will cough a lot less.
2. You will have more energy – Within 2 to 12 weeks, blood circulation improves dramatically, giving you much more energy to exercise and look after yourself. The physical activity we looked at earlier will be easy.
3. You will be less stressed – Studies have shown that by quitting smoking, your stress levels will greatly decrease. If you suffer from stress, you will find that quitting smoking will help and offer more natural ways to manage your stress.
4. You will have better sex – For men, stopping smoking will improve erections. For women, orgasms improve and arousal becomes easier.
5. You will be more fertile – By becoming a non-smoker, your chance of conceiving a child, naturally or via IVF, is increased.

6. Your smell and taste improve – Smoking dulls your taste buds and blunts your sense of smell. You will be surprised by what you will begin to smell and taste!

7. You will look younger – Quitting smoking will improve your skin. The skin of non-smokers gets more nutrients and receives more oxygen.

8. Your teeth will be whiter – The tobacco in smoke stains your teeth a yellow colour. By stopping smoking, you will also have fresher breath.

9. You will live longer – Half of all long-term smokers die younger from smoking-related diseases (heart disease, lung cancer and chronic bronchitis).

10. You will protect your loved ones – When you stop smoking, you will be protecting your family and loved ones. Studies have shown that second-hand smoke is seriously dangerous.

There is also a very popular and effective NHS Smokefree app on the One You website. If you struggle to stop, keep trying. Never give up hope. The journey is long, but in the end you will eventually stop and you will feel much better. Many people find the NHS Stop Smoking service helpful as it gives the extra support they need, and studies show that you are four times more likely to quit smoking if you do it through the NHS Stop Smoking service. You can make an appointment without first seeing your GP by calling the NHS Stop Smoking helpline and you can find the number to call on the NHS Choices website. A Stop Smoking adviser will give you advice, support and the drugs that are available to reduce the cravings – nicotine replacement therapy (NRT), buproprion (Zyban) and varenicline (Champix). If you prefer, you can ask your GP to make the referral to the NHS Stop Smoking service but many GPs like to provide personal support themselves and can of course prescribe NRT or the supportive drugs.

For some people, e-cigarettes have been helpful in stopping smoking and Public Health England supported them in a major report in 2015. At present, it seems that they are less harmful than tobacco cigarettes but taking any new chemical into your body should always be done with caution if no one knows the effect of the long-term use of the substance. Simply switching to e-cigarettes and using them long-term is therefore not as sensible as using them to try to stop smoking tobacco cigarettes as a short-term measure. More research will clarify the risks and benefits of e-cigarettes and reduce the disagreement between expert groups, but in 2016 the Royal College of Physicians released a report stating that it 'believes that e-cigarettes could lead to significant falls in the prevalence of smoking in the UK, prevent many deaths and episodes of serious illness, and help to reduce the social inequalities in health that tobacco smoking currently exacerbates'.

Don't let past failures put you off – quit smoking. The benefits are great not only in terms of preventing diseases such as lung cancer and heart disease but in helping people who already have a health problem feel better. People with chronic obstructive pulmonary disease (bronchitis) or asthma, for example, will benefit from stopping smoking. As the British Lung Foundation emphasises, 'It's never too late to give up!'

Resources on smoking	What's in it for you
Health Check	You will be asked if you smoke, encouraged to try quitting again if you have tried before and referred to the NHS Stop Smoking service
One You	The How Are You quiz will ask how many cigarettes you smoke daily and send you a stop smoking programme

(continued)

Resources on smoking	What's in it for you
Your annual review if you have a long-term condition like type 2 diabetes or high blood pressure	You should be asked about smoking and given support to try to stop smoking but it may not happen, in which case search for 'stop smoking' in NHS Choices
NHS Choices	You can get help from the NHS Stop Smoking service
High-quality apps	Try http://quitnow.smokefree.nhs.uk

Your gut, bowels and liver

Digestive complaints and issues are very common and are treatable, most of the time, by over-the-counter medicines. Around 40 per cent of people have at least one digestive symptom at any one time. The most common are:

- changes in bowel movement (constipation or diarrhoea)
- heartburn
- indigestion

These can usually be treated with the lifestyle changes which we've already discussed – diet and exercise. The medicine from the pharmacy should be a short-term fix, and if the symptoms persist you should consider visiting your GP.

To help ease your digestive movements, the message is simple:

- Eat Mediterranean to keep your weight steady or reduce it. It is important to keep your guts and bowels in good working order.
- Fill up on fibre – for a healthy bowel, you need fibre from a variety of sources (wholemeal bread, fruit, vegetables, beans and oats).

- Drink plenty of fluid to aid digestion.
- Try to avoid eating too much spice as this can upset your stomach.
- Drink less alcohol – use the online checker in NHS Choices to compare how much you drink with what research says is high-risk drinking and, at 50, consider building two alcohol-free days into your week.

Your skin

Your skin is the largest organ. It protects you, heals you and makes you feel confident. It is also one of the most obvious signs of ageing. It is the thing everyone (including yourself) will notice. Your skin keeps you healthy so the least you can do is take care of it. Women aged 40 and over are usually right on top of this, sometimes at unnecessary expense. For men, and for women too, there are a few simple rules:

- There is no strong scientific evidence that anything labelled as 'anti-ageing' has any significant effect on skin ageing other than through the cream in which the so-called anti-ageing element is dissolved.
- Use a simple, inexpensive aqueous cream liberally, all over. Try to moisturise every day, or at least once a week.
- Protect your skin from excessive ultraviolet light from the sun. Some people are probably as tanned as they want to be at 50 and should now reduce their risk of the type of skin cancer called melanoma. So use strong sun protection, factor 15 or 30, and take 25μg of vitamin D a day to compensate for the fact that sun cream will stop your skin making enough of this vitamin. Many people who live in the United

Kingdom are deficient in vitamin D, and this makes bones thinner. If you can't make sufficient vitamin D naturally because your sunscreen is blocking the sun's rays then a tablet a day prevents this deficiency.

On top of this, you should stop smoking, as that greatly harms your skin. Smoking reduces the blood flow to your skin, making you look older and more ill. Similarly, excessive drinking of alcohol will dehydrate your skin, leaving you looking older and tired. Drinking water will keep your skin hydrated and prevent it drying out.

The Harvard Medical School Special Health Report 'Skin Care and Repair' debunks ten myths about skin care. They are:

1. The right skin cream can keep your skin looking young.
2. Antibacterial soap is best for keeping your skin clean.
3. Eating chocolate or oily foods causes oily skin and acne.
4. Tanning is bad for you.
5. Tanning is good for you.
6. The higher the SPF of your sunscreen, the better.
7. A scar that is barely noticeable is the mark of a good surgeon.
8. Vitamin E will make scars fade.
9. Crossing your legs causes varicose veins.
10. Scalp massage can prevent baldness.

So don't believe all you read, and keep your skin-care routine simple.

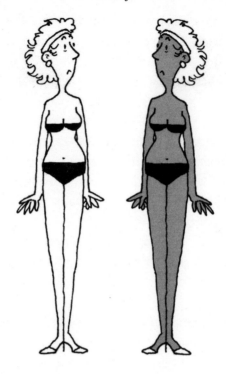

Your bones, joints and muscles

For both bones and muscles the advice is the same: they will become stronger using the training for strength techniques described in Part Three. Every exercise that makes your muscles stronger will strengthen the bones, and every exercise that strengthens your muscles will help them support your joints better, but for joints the most important aspect of fitness is suppleness. From 40 on you need a daily routine built on the principles of one of the four great suppleness programmes, yoga, tai chi, Pilates and the Alexander technique.

Women should also ensure they drink a pint of milk a day, or eat enough calcium-rich foods if milk is not palatable, and although the experts are not in universal agreement, taking

25μg of vitamin D daily is probably sensible, but the exercise is more important.

Your metabolism

Your metabolism is your engine. It converts the potential energy in what you eat to the actual energy that your body needs – for your muscles, obviously, but also for your brain, your liver and every living tissue.

If you put too much energy into yourself, however, it will turn into fat, more easily in some people than others, probably for genetic reasons, but it will happen to everyone. Another problem occurs if you do this year after year. Your pancreas, a gland which acts like an energy thermostat, switching on insulin production when blood sugar levels go up, becomes exhausted and run down – just as a battery will run down if you leave the car lights on all the time. When this happens the pancreas fails to produce enough insulin. The result is that the person develops what some people call the metabolic syndrome, which is a combination of type 2 diabetes, high blood pressure and obesity. Decreased expenditure of energy is at least as much to blame for the epidemics of obesity and type 2 diabetes as the increase of energy intake.

Unfortunately, humans do not have anything as remotely useful and accurate as the mounting price of petrol shown on the pump at your filling station. What you need to do is to learn how to judge the amount of energy you are taking in and how much you are using, as described in Part Four.

Your teeth and gums

From the age of 40, you need to focus your energy on your gums. From childhood the emphasis is all on teeth and tooth brushing, and rightly so. But when you are in midlife with a full set of teeth, or almost a full set, you need to think ahead. The danger to your teeth and to your bank balance comes not from the teeth themselves but from the gums.

Unless you start to look after your gums as well as your teeth obsessively, the teeth are doomed. The teeth can stay healthy, brushed twice a day and perfectly filled or crowned, but they will simply come loose and fall out of gums that have not been properly looked after. What happens is shown below.

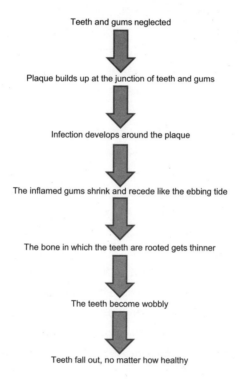

Teeth and gums neglected

Plaque builds up at the junction of teeth and gums

Infection develops around the plaque

The inflamed gums shrink and recede like the ebbing tide

The bone in which the teeth are rooted gets thinner

The teeth become wobbly

Teeth fall out, no matter how healthy

So you need to care of both teeth and gums in two ways – eat well and brush well.

Let's look at your diet first. Sugar is just as damaging to the teeth of adults as it is to the teeth of children. You should therefore eat as little sugar as you can, as few times a day as possible.

Remember that sugar in fruit can be as bad as the refined sugar in the obvious sources. If you eat grapes or a banana between meals instead of a high-calorie snack, remember to try to clean some of the surplus sugar off the surface of your teeth, even a mini gargle with some water is good if you can. Try to stick to three meals a day and after each meal clean your teeth as well as you can. If you can, brush them; if you can't, rinse out your mouth with water. Some dentists with a particular interest in preventive dentistry for adults recommend sugarless chewing gum too, because it cruises about the mouth picking up the crumbs that would lead to plaque, and some artificial sweeteners may also help protect the teeth and gums from a build-up of plaque.

Now, let's look at brushing. You need to spend at least five minutes a night on your teeth and gums. Many of us have enjoyed that technological wonder the electric toothbrush for years, assuming it was all we needed, but it has its deficiencies. The rotation buffs up the teeth but only on their surface. You need to dig deeper. Here's what to do:

- Use a special little pointy brush, called an interspace brush, to clean between your teeth, taking about a minute to go round the top and bottom. Push it up and down hard on the line where the gums meet the teeth.
- Next use dental floss, not in and out but up and down between the teeth. Try to picture the floss sliding down the edge of each tooth and then pressing down on the gum.
- Use a special little brush, called an interdental brush, to push through the junctions between teeth and gums.
- Use an ordinary old-fashioned manual toothbrush for another attack on the junction between tooth and gum. Focus particularly on the lower teeth because plaque grows faster there. Brush downwards on both the insides and the outsides.

- Now finish off with the electric toothbrush, but remember that it only cleans the surface of the teeth – like polishing the outside of the car but leaving the interior full of sandwich wrappers, apple cores and little bits of biscuit – unless it is one of the newer brushes, such as the Philips Sonicare range, that vibrate and attack the borderland between teeth and gums.

This should take at least five minutes and you can get even more value by standing on one leg while doing this work. It is very good training to keep up your balancing skills!

The 'manopause'

Type 'buy testosterone' into Google and you get a number of responses; type in 'Low T' and you get even more! If you pick on a typical Low T or low testosterone website, it tells you the symptoms are:

- fatigue
- weakness
- depression
- sleep disturbances

Of course the one you would expect is there too, but many of the personal testimonies that populate these sites talk of a 'loss of desire' rather than inability to 'get it up' when there is ardent desire. Loss of desire or even diminished desire could, like all the other symptoms listed above, equally well be caused by loss of fitness, or could be the consequence of depression. For these reasons most of the medical profession does not consider there to be a male equivalent of the menopause, sometimes ridiculously called the 'manopause', even though sales of testosterone are huge and increasing, mainly in the USA, with new 'Low T clinics' opening in many countries.

There is no doubt that some men suffer from severe testosterone deficiency, for example as a result of testicular disease, but the evidence for prescribing or buying testosterone is weak. There was great excitement in January 2016 when all the media carried reports of research about the benefits of testosterone, but a closer examination of the paper that caused all the furore when it was published in Volume 374 of the prestigious *New England Journal of Medicine* reveals a more cautious conclusion, indeed that very common conclusion – further research is needed. Here is the conclusion of Professor Peter J. Snyder's study:

> In symptomatic men 65 years of age or older, raising testosterone concentrations for 1 year from moderately low to the mid-normal range for men 19 to 40 years of age had a moderate benefit with respect to sexual function and some benefit with respect to mood and depressive symptoms but no benefit with respect to vitality or walking distance. The number of participants was too few to draw conclusions about the risks of testosterone treatment.

For all the symptoms said to be caused by 'Low T', try getting fitter, not testosterone, unless there is some medical or surgical reason for testosterone deficiency.

The menopause

It is relatively easy to provide information to people with heart disease or cancer. The course the disease follows is relatively, but only relatively, similar in everybody and so too are the actions that need to be considered at each stage of the disease. This is not the case with the menopause which is a normal biological process that varies very much from one person to another.

There are some generalisations that can be made: for example, the meanings of the terms 'menopause' and 'perimenopause', which are spelled out in the guidance produced by NICE. This guidance, which is written for both doctors and women, is clear and easy to read – search for NICE and menopause online.

There is now agreement that there are two conditions – the perimenopause and the menopause. The term perimenopause is used to describe a condition in which there are irregular periods and symptoms like hot flushes, with the menopause defined as not having had a period for 12 months. The perimenopause itself can last for 4 to 8 years.

The guidance emphasises that treatment has to be individualised for a number of reasons, not only because the symptoms and distress of the perimenopause and menopause vary very much from one woman to another. The other key factor is that the treatments on offer are themselves not without side effects and every person has to decide how they feel about the possible risks as well as the possible benefits.

As always, before going to see your GP or a specialist take time to think about, and write down, what is bothering you most and read the section on the menopause in NHS Choices. Be prepared to discuss what is important to you, in order to improve your quality of life during the consultation.

3

Your Health Services

As I said earlier, health care is what you do for yourself to stay healthy, reduce the risk of disease and ensure that any condition you do develop has minimal impact on your well-being and vitality. Health services are provided by the NHS and by local authorities to help you with your health care and there are many services that have been mentioned throughout this book.

The mission of the NHS is to prevent, diagnose and treat disease but the prevention of disease depends on many factors other than the NHS. For example, the prevention of heart disease also depends on what the government does to help people stop smoking. Prevention also depends on what you do for yourself. But there are things the NHS can do to help you reduce your risk and there are four risk-reduction programmes that are available free:

- NHS Choices – your knowledge service
- the One You programme – your online health improvement and support service
- the NHS Health Check programme – your risk assessment service
- the Annual Health Review – your personal support service if you already have a long-term problem and therefore won't be offered a Health Check

The aim of all these services is to help you feel better and reduce the risk of serious health problems, particularly the two most common physical problems:

- Cancer (and there are also screening programmes for common cancers)
- Heart disease, stroke and dementia

In addition, the One You programme has been designed to help lower the risk of long-term mental health problems by reducing the effects of stress, and NHS Choices also contains many resources designed to improve mental health and reduce the risk of the most common of all chronic health problems – mental illness.

NHS choices

Knowledge is the enemy of disease. Clean, clear, accessible knowledge is as important for your health in the 21st century as clean, clear water was in the 19th century.

NHS Choices (www.nhs.uk) is a knowledge service that contains all the information you need – based on the best research, interviews with people (real people as well as experts), tips on how to deal with stress or stop smoking, and programmes to help you sleep better or eat better – all designed for your phone when you have very little time to spare. It was designed to give you, the citizen, access to the best current medical knowledge, the best evidence that is available. All that is missing is direct access to all the journals that doctors can consult in a medical library, but that is not a great loss. Research has shown that a goodly proportion of the medical research that is published is shown to be untrue within a year; NHS Choices is designed to provide knowledge that has been distilled to improve its strength and quality.

Health issues commonly make headlines, often dramatic headlines, with claims such as 'Rhubarb cure for dementia!' You need to be careful and remember that there are two types of newspaper articles. Firstly, there is the news story, sometimes written by the newspaper's health correspondent. However, many front-page stories are written by someone who happened to be on the news desk when a press release arrived. It is also important to remember that, when the story has been written, the headline is usually added afterwards by a subeditor keen to make it dramatic in order to catch the attention of the passer-by. For this reason, the NHS Choices website has a service called 'Behind the Headlines' in which, within a day, the stories behind the blockbuster headlines are analysed. 'Behind the Headlines' found that although it was usual to lay blame at the door of the journalist who wrote the story, the hype usually emanated from the press release produced by the academic researcher seeking more money for research, or the company seeking investment and profit.

The other source of information in newspapers comes from their health sections or supplements, which often appear on a Tuesday in the *Daily Mail* and the *Daily Express*, for example. These articles are written by journalists who have special-ised in writing about health, and some of them are medically qualified – the 'media medics'. Their reporting is usually well balanced and helpful, so it is worth reading the health sections in your newspaper regularly, and even keeping an eye open for those in other newspapers perhaps discarded at work.

The best place to start if you want clear information about a particular topic is the NHS Choices website: www.nhs.uk

The one you programme

One You (www.nhs.uk/oneyou) is an online programme which offers you the opportunity to review your health risks through its How Are You quiz. It gives you personalised information and links to both local and online services, including apps, that can help you reduce those risks.

This is a great new programme which takes the NHS for the first time into using your phone to help you reduce your risk of disease.

The NHS health check programme

The NHS Health Check programme was introduced to give people over 40 who have no reason to have regular contact with the NHS the chance to assess their health risks:

Do you have or have you had:

- Heart disease or a 20 per cent risk of developing it
- Chronic kidney disease
- Diabetes (type 1 or type 2)
- Hypertension (a fancy name for high blood pressure)
- Atrial fibrillation (irregular pulse)
- Hypercholesterolaemia (high levels of cholesterol in your blood) or currently being prescribed statins
- Heart failure
- Peripheral arterial disease (narrowing of the arteries in the leg leading to muscle pain when walking)
- Stroke or transient ischaemic attack (TIA) – sometimes called a mini-stroke

No: You will receive an invitation for an NHS Health Check every five years.

Yes: You will not get an invitation for an NHS Health Check but you will get an annual health review

---

Health Checks are organised by your local council and are available either through Health Check clinics or in your own health centre or a local pharmacy. The aim of the NHS Health

Check is to give you knowledge both about risk and about your-self, to help you review your health and lifestyle and identify steps that could be taken to reduce your risk of serious disease later on. The process varies a little from one place to another but there are some elements always present, namely:

- A questionnaire about your lifestyle, but you should use the How Are You quiz before you go for your NHS Health Check: it gets your mind in gear.
- An assessment of your height and weight, pulse rate and blood pressure by a practice nurse or health-care assistant.
- A blood test of your blood fats, blood sugar and kidney function.

The most important element is not the blood test but the conversation with the health-care assistant and the opportunity to reflect afterwards on issues that have been identified for you to think about.

The annual health review

If you are a person who is ineligible for a Health Check because you have a condition like atrial fibrillation, then you should be invited at least once a year for a review by your hospital specialist or GP. (Remember, too, that your pharmacist is an excellent source of advice if you are taking medication for a long-term condition, and they know about health risks as well as about drugs.) This review, which should be a comprehensive assessment of all your risk factors, should also evaluate the progress of your condition and the effectiveness of the treatment. These reviews are not as well organised as the Health Checks, so the busy clinician may not have time to cover all the risk factors. Perhaps the best first step you can take is to complete the How Are You quiz before you go to the clinic because there is now strong scientific evidence that people with conditions such as type 2 diabetes would benefit just as much as, if not more than, people who do not have disease from reducing stress, increasing activity, eating less 'crap', quitting smoking and sleeping better. Such advice is as important as the drugs the doctor prescribes.

Coping better with stress, getting fitter and eating better are at least as important to people who have developed heart disease, or any other disease or condition, as to those people who do not have a disease.

This applies to all people with long-term health problems, including cancer. The wonderful charity Macmillan Cancer Support has done great work, not only emphasising the importance of a good diet and exercise but organising health walks in partnership with the Ramblers, in a campaign called Walking for Health.

Reducing the risk of cancer by screening

The purpose of screening is to identify disease before the disease causes symptoms, providing it has been proved in research that the detection of disease at that stage is likely to do more good than harm. It might seem self-evident that finding disease earlier would always be a good idea and at one time there was great enthusiasm in the medical profession for screening. However, we now know that not everyone who has what seem like early signs of disease, but no symptoms, will develop that disease. The big problem is that an increase in survival does not necessarily prove that screening is effective; it could be due to something called lead time bias.

We also know that screening, like all medical care, can have harmful side effects, so the medical profession is now much more cautious about screening. Some people feel that screening has been oversold by the NHS and Public Health England, namely that the benefits have been overplayed and the risks and harms underplayed, because screening can do harm: it can create anxiety and lead to investigations or treatments that themselves carry a risk. The NHS and Public Health England are, however, cautious in deciding which cancers to screen for and emphasise on the National Screening Committee website that 'screening is different to diagnosis and there will always be some false positive and false negative results'. So, consider the invitation to have a screening test as an opportunity to reduce your risk of disease but be very cautious about accepting invitations for private screening, or even offers of free screening at work.

Reducing the risk of breast and cervical cancer by screening

For women in their forties and fifties there is screening for cervical cancer. The cervical screening programme, like all screening programmes, misses some cancers so some women will die of cervical cancer if they have had a negative smear test with what is called a false negative result – that is, the smear test is negative but the woman is developing a cancer. This is an inevitable part of all screening programmes which have both false negative results and false positive results – a positive screening test leading to treatment for a condition that would never develop into a cancer that would kill or even become apparent in the life of the individual.

There is more debate about the benefits and limitations of breast cancer screening. Like all decisions, the decision about whether or not to accept the invitation for screening has to be determined by your personal values as well as by the scientific evidence. The evidence is:

- Mammography and follow-up assessment and treatment of the cancers detected reduce the risk of dying from breast cancer.
- A number of women will have cancers detected that will not progress and would have remained undetected without causing harm if they had not accepted the offer of screening.

The NHS Choices website sets out the benefits and the risks, particularly the risk of overtreatment, emphasising that 'some women who have screening will be diagnosed and treated for breast cancer that would never otherwise have caused them harm'. Screening is a risk-reduction activity and the choice is personal. Women are offered this opportunity for reducing the risk of dying from breast cancer. Screening is offered to all women over the age of 50 and in some parts of the country to women aged 47 to 49 as part of a research project to find out if screening under the age of 50 is worthwhile.

Reducing the risk of bowel cancer by screening

Screening for bowel cancer has been offered to people aged over 60 for about ten years. The test that is used looks for traces of blood in the faeces, but now a new test is being introduced for people aged 55, who will be offered a single once-in-a-lifetime test. Called the bowel scope test, it involves passing a flexible tube called a flexible sigmoidoscope into the lower part of your large bowel from the bottom upwards – it sounds worse than it is! This allows the identification of little growths called polyps, which can usually be snipped off. To learn more, look at NHS Choices.

Reducing the risk of other cancers by screening

- Ovarian cancer

Although there have been promising results from research into screening for ovarian cancer, the experts are divided and at present there is no screening programme.

- Lung cancer

There are also some promising early results of screening for lung cancer in people at very high risk, however the evidence is not considered strong enough to introduce a screening programme. Unlike ovarian cancer however there is one sure way of reducing the risk of this type of cancer – stop smoking.

- Prostate cancer

The problem of the false positive is even more difficult in screening for prostate cancer and this has been, and continues to be, a very hot topic. Here are the key facts:

- False positives are a particular problem in PSA testing for prostate cancer.
- If you examine the prostates of healthy men, many of them will have clumps of cells that look exactly like the cells you see in a cancer that has spread and will be fatal.
- However, not all of the cancers that are seen will develop into cancers that will cause problems or kill.
- The PSA test finds all cancers, the ones that will kill and the ones that will never cause any trouble.
- By looking down a microscope it is not possible to tell which cancers will kill and which will not.
- The treatment for prostate cancer will leave some men incontinent or impotent, or both, even in the best of cancer treatment services.

For this reason the NHS does not offer PSA screening to men under 60 because there is no evidence that it will reduce the risk of dying from prostate cancer. If you are worried about prostate cancer you can find more information about PSA testing and reducing your risk of prostate cancer on NHS Choices. Interestingly, a study from Oxford University reported that there was a significant reduction in risk of prostate cancer among men who had reduced their waist size in trousers! Whether it was the weight loss itself, or the change in diet and exercise, is not clear, but as with many cancers what is emerging is the fact that our modern environment increases the risk of cancer in the population and that there are genetic factors in some cancers that determine which people in the population will develop cancer. Undoubtedly better tests will be developed, probably based on the genes that determine which of the cellular changes that take place are going to develop into cancers that kill and which will remain in the prostate until you die of something else.

Spend your hard earned money on fitness, not private screening

It is now accepted that a car should have regular servicing, and that it must have an MOT once a year, but what about your body? Is it not advisable to check the petrol, the oil and the tire pressure regularly? The answer is yes, so you need to look after your body too, but regular servicing by someone else can cause problems.

When the garage says 'the battery is on its last legs' or 'you are going to have trouble with the front tires this winter', it is difficult to argue. After all, they are the experts. But they may be wrong. Even worse than the unnecessary expenditure that may follow this type of gloomy report, new problems can be actually caused by overenthusiastic servicing.

Medical tests can do harm as well as good, principally from what is now called 'overdiagnosis', for example from blood test results that are not quite 'normal' – a term that most doctors do not use any more – or x-ray or MRI images they don't understand but feel they have to report by saying something like 'the possibility of cancer could not be excluded'. For this reason, you should not envy top executives who are given annual check-ups; they may do more harm than good and are avoided by the great majority of doctors.

In this book we have described the health and prevention services offered by the NHS and the public health services, both nationally from Public Health England and locally from your local council. These services (such as One You, the NHS Health Check and NHS Choices) are important, but healthcare is something you do for yourself, supported by the NHS and there are other health services which are very important.

Reducing your risk of heart disease, stroke and dementia

For decades press interest has switched from blood pressure to cholesterol to obesity and back again as the various experts argue that the risk factor in which they are most interested is the most important. What is now clear is that, not surprisingly, all these risk factors are interrelated and that it is the overall level of risk that is important, rather than any single factor. Common sense, really. For example an imbalance between food consumption (energy intake) and energy expenditure leads to an increase in weight, which not only raises the blood pressure and cholesterol but also often reduces the amount of energy used, which further increases the weight gain and so on and so on. Obviously cigarette smoking stands on its own, but it is now also added into an overall estimate of risk.

The NHS Health Check uses a formula called the QRisk2

cardiovascular risk score which brings together all the different risk factors into a single score that tells you your risk of having a 'cardiovascular event' – that is, a stroke or heart attack – and expresses your risk in the following way:

Your QRisk2 score	What it means for you
10% or less	Among 100 people like you, fewer than 10 will have a heart attack or stroke in the next 10 years
10.1% to 19.9%	Among 100 people like you, more than 10 but fewer than 20 will have a heart attack or stroke in the next 10 years
20% or more	Among 100 people like you, at least 20 will have a heart attack or stroke in the next 10 years

It is also now clear that the risk of that condition which many people dread even more than cancer can also be reduced by the same steps as those that reduce the risk of heart disease, because a common cause of dementia is the same disease of the small arteries that causes heart attacks, a disease called atherosclerosis.

You can also carry out your own risk assessment by using the heart age tool on NHS Choices. This is easy to use and good fun if you share the result with friends.

Reducing the risk from obesity and type 2 diabetes

Earlier, we looked at measuring your body mass index (BMI). Your NHS Health Check will do the same. It will come as no surprise to be told your BMI is high and you are overweight or obese, because you can see that in your mirror! There is no real difference between being overweight and being obese – it is all a matter of risk, and the higher your BMI, the higher your risk.

Another reason for assessing the BMI is that it indicates the average level of your blood sugar better than a single blood sample because the level of glucose in your blood goes down and up very markedly before and after a meal or snack. This may lead the nurse or GP to tell you that you have the metabolic syndrome, pre-diabetes, or type 2 diabetes.

The term metabolic syndrome is not helpful. It simply means that you have been taking in more energy than you need for years, and your pancreas, which produces the insulin that reduces your blood sugar, is getting exhausted and is not working very well. Similarly, pre-diabetes is a new term that is also controversial and many doctors do not use it because it is not a disease and it also simply means that for years you have been taking more energy than you need, and your pancreas is now getting exhausted and is not working too well – much the same as the metabolic syndrome.

If you are told you have type 2 diabetes, this does not mean that you have suddenly developed a disease like tuberculosis. Again, it means that for many years you have been taking in more energy than you need and your pancreas is now exhausted and no longer able to produce enough insulin. This means not only that you need to cut down energy intake, for example by eating less sugar, and increase your energy expenditure by taking more exercise, but also that you need to take a pill or two every day. Some doctors wait a month or two to see if the blood sugar comes down and prescribe exercise and a change in diet rather than prescribing medication immediately, because type 2 diabetes is a curable condition. Discuss this option with your GP. Most people, however, will need a pill or two for the rest of their lives, but even more important is to adapt to the shock of diagnosis and develop a new approach to life. In addition to the help from your GP and practice nurse, there is good information and support on both the NHS Choices and Diabetes UK websites and the first step is not to take a pill but to increase exercise and eat a better balanced diet with less calories. As the Diabetes UK website states *'sometimes diet and exercise are not enough to control Type 2 Diabetes and you may need to take diabetes medication'*.

The NHS, Public Health England and Diabetes UK launched a major diabetes prevention campaign in 2015. Type 1 diabetes is a disease of unknown cause, which starts out of the blue, but type 2 diabetes is a condition caused by our environment. Look back over Part Three of this book for ways to increase your exercise regime.

By adapting to the challenges of 21st-century life type 2 diabetes can be prevented or, if it develops, the complications can be prevented by changes in the way you live, sometimes helped by prescribed drugs. This is the aim of the NHS campaign now called Healthier You. The challenge of type 2 diabetes for the individual affected and for the population as a whole demonstrates the need to think in a new way about health and disease. In the old days we gave people who were healthy, by which we meant they had not had any disease or condition diagnosed, information and advice on exercise and good eating; people who had had a diagnosis of type 2 diabetes or high blood pressure or depression were given pills and other forms of treatment delivered by doctors and other clinicians. Now we know that people who have had a disease or condition diagnosed need advice and support to encourage exercise and good eating at least as much as people who have not yet developed a condition.

The diagnosis of a condition like type 2 diabetes is not a death sentence. It is potentially curable. It does not condemn you to a life of pill-taking and depression. Better to regard it as a wake-up call encouraging you to adopt a new approach to life and take care of yourself better. Once you have a long-term condition diagnosed you need to reduce your risks of other disease and complications and we now know that activities that were previously thought to be preventive, such as exercise, are very, very important as part of the treatment of diseases like heart disease and type 2 diabetes.

Reducing the risk from high blood pressure

The term 'high blood pressure' implies that there is a disease called high blood pressure and that you either have it or you don't. In practice there is no sharp cut-off between what is called high blood pressure and normal blood pressure. Everyone has blood pressure – if they don't, they are dead! Some people, however, have a level of blood pressure that puts them at increased risk of kidney disease, stroke and heart disease, and what the doctors should say is 'You have a level of blood pressure which is higher than average and which increases your risk of a stroke, heart disease and dementia to such a degree that we recommend taking drugs to lower your blood pressure, even though the drugs cause side effects in a proportion of people.' This is, however, a bit longer than the simple statement 'You have high blood pressure', so that is what is usually said.

In 2014, the NHS and Public Health England, working with three key charities – Blood Pressure UK, the British Heart Foundation, and the British Hypertension Society – launched a campaign called 'Tackling High Blood Pressure'. This aims firstly to get more people aware of their blood pressure, therefore identifying more people who would benefit from lowering it. Secondly, it aims to help people lower their blood pressure by:

- reducing salt intake
- reducing weight
- increasing activity levels

The British Heart Foundation, the leading heart disease charity, is equally clear. Their very helpful website states: *'If your doctor or nurse says you have high blood pressure, they are likely to encourage you to make some lifestyle changes to help reduce it. This may include increasing your physical activity, losing weight, reducing the salt in your diet, cutting down on alcohol and eating a balanced, healthy diet. If your blood pressure is very high or these lifestyle changes do not reduce it enough, your doctor is likely to prescribe you medication.'*

A major NHS and Public Health England campaign to tackle high blood pressure and prevent its complications was launched in 2014, however, the most important person in tackling high blood pressure is you.

Reducing the risk from atrial fibrillation

In checking your blood pressure the nurse will also note if the rhythm is regular or irregular. If the pulse is irregular, the condition is called atrial fibrillation; the word atrial refers to the part of the heart where its natural pacemaker is situated and the word fibrillation means fluttering. Atrial fibrillation is a very important risk factor for stroke and dementia because blood clots form in the heart if it is not beating regularly and shoot off to the brain. Fortunately, the condition can be treated with anticoagulant drugs.

Reducing the risk from high cholesterol

The level of cholesterol in your blood is a bit like your blood pressure. It is a risk factor. Everyone has cholesterol in their blood – vegetarians and vegans as well as people who consume meat daily. High cholesterol itself doesn't usually cause any symptoms, but it can increase your risk of serious health conditions down the line. Cholesterol can restrict blood flow to your heart, your brain and the rest of your body. Your risk of developing coronary heart disease also rises as your blood's cholesterol increases.

If, during your health check, you're told that your cholesterol is raised then the first thing to remember is not to panic. High cholesterol won't kill you tomorrow. Regard it as a risk factor, something that tells you that action is needed.

The first step in reducing your cholesterol is to have a healthy and balanced diet. See Part Four for the correct foods you should be eating. Swap food containing saturated fat and start eating more fruit, vegetables and wholegrain cereals. As I've mentioned, the Mediterranean diet is a great example to follow. Here are a few other tips:

- Replace butter, lard and ghee with unsaturated oils from plants and seeds such as olive and rapeseed oil.
- Eat oily fish, such as mackerel, salmon and tuna.
- Fibre, found in wholegrain rice, bread and pasta, has also been shown to help lower cholesterol.
- Instead of frying your food, try grilling, steaming or poaching.
- Choose lean cuts of meat and go for lower-fat varieties of dairy products and spreads.

The next step in reducing your cholesterol is to exercise more. Being active, as we have discovered, will help you maintain a healthy weight, or lose weight if you're overweight. Being overweight increases the amount of 'bad cholesterol' in your blood. If you need another benefit for doing more exercise, then physical activity will help lower your blood pressure and it will keep your heart and blood vessels in working order. Take a look at Part Three of this book for the activities you can take part in.

Coping with a long-term condition

From the age of 40 on, health problems become more common. Many of them are preventable by the techniques and methods described in this book, but by the age of 40, nearly 40 per cent of people have at least one medical problem, rising to 50 per cent by the age of 50. Sometimes the problem is a disease but it is often what doctors call a 'long-term condition'.

Doctors have been diagnosing diseases for centuries. Some diseases are acute and they come on quickly with symptoms. Appendicitis and heart attacks are examples of acute diseases. Other diseases such as asthma, epilepsy or rheumatoid arthritis are chronic or long-term. People with chronic diseases usually get on with their lives without seeking to be recognised as being ill. In fact, they may have to convince people that they are still fully able to do a job and should not be sidelined for promotion or made redundant just because they have developed some long-term or chronic disease.

Some long-term diseases are only too obvious to the person affected – depression or arthritis, for example – but medical testing reveals a new set of conditions which do not cause symptoms, such as high blood pressure, atrial fibrillation and type 2 diabetes.

These conditions are often without any symptoms and are therefore discovered by accident when you visit the doctor for another reason or as part of a health check, either by the NHS or at work.

When you get the diagnosis of a disease or a long-term condition, it has a psychological, and sometimes physical, impact. For example, if you develop arthritis you may find it more difficult to take exercise and this leads to a loss of fitness which will widen the fitness gap. Unfortunately, sometimes people who develop long-term health problems do not receive the right advice about staying active. (This can be complicated by well-meaning relatives and friends who think it kinder to do things for a person who obviously has difficulty instead of helping that person to find ways of doing the job themselves.) In such circumstances fitness is lost even more quickly than can be explained by the direct effects of the disease.

Not surprisingly, people who have more than one physical problem often develop mental health problems too. Anxiety or depression can be a consequence of suddenly being told that you have one or more conditions that have no symptoms, but which increase the risk of early death or disability. A vicious cycle can develop.

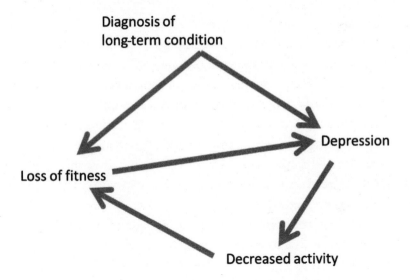

However, what we know now is that people who develop long-term diseases and conditions have even more need to focus on stopping smoking, getting fitter, eating better and sleeping better than people without these diagnoses.

In comparison, those people who have a positive attitude in response to their diagnosis, and view it as a wake-up call, will reduce their risk of complications and will feel better; let's call it a 'virtuous cycle'.

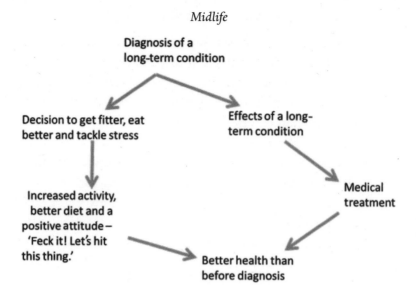

Diagnosis of a long-term condition

Decision to get fitter, eat better and tackle stress

Effects of a long-term condition

Increased activity, better diet and a positive attitude – 'Feck it! Let's hit this thing.'

Medical treatment

Better health than before diagnosis

For example, if you are told you have a condition such as type 2 diabetes, the attention is too often on the drug treatment of the condition. The complexity of diet management and drug therapy is very time-consuming but as Diabetes UK emphasises, it is vitally important for people with type 2 diabetes to stop smoking, eat better, sleep well and get fitter. Everything in this book about reducing the risk of disease or getting fitter is of even more importance to those of you who have had a long-term condition identified.

It is also very important to be cautious about offers of treatments to make sure the decision is right for you.

Making the treatment decision that is right for you

The NHS is a wonderful thing and it is very comforting for people in midlife who are starting to make more use of the NHS, or have parents who are now receiving a lot of help from the NHS, to have access to health services without fear of debt or bankruptcy. However it is very important to understand that health services can do harm as well as good.

The term 'patient' implies someone who sits quietly and does what their doctor recommends but it is now accepted, by the medical profession, that it is essential for the person who is seeking help from the NHS to be equally active in making decisions about their health.

Before you go and see the doctor, make sure you are clear about what is really bothering you. Then, if the doctor diagnoses a disease, ask:

- 'Will treatment of this disease make a difference to what is bothering me most?'

Then, if treatment will make a difference, ask:

- 'If 1,000 people with a problem like mine are treated, what number will benefit?'
- 'If 1,000 people with a problem like mine are treated, what number will be harmed?'

Advances in health technology have made a huge difference to the health of people in every developed country. Hip replacement, cancer treatment, transplantation and stents for heart disease are wonderful developments but there is growing concern about the adverse effects of technology, particularly when it is offered to people who are not seriously ill. The press, the public and the medical profession and researchers have focused on the benefits of health service technology in the last 50 years but growing attention is now focused on the harm that medical care can cause and therefore on the balance of good to harm.

If you are being offered a treatment with serious side effects – an operation, for example – you should be given a Patient Decision Aid, namely a web-based service to help you really think through the options of accepting or declining the offer of treatment. There is good-quality information available about all the options and the health problems of a particular treatment. Using a Decision Aid will help you make an informed decision about which option is best for you and what option suits you best. For more information about a treatment go to the NHS Choices website and type the name of your treatment and 'decision aid' into the search engine. For more information about overdiagnosis look at the BMJ website www.bmj.com and type 'overdiagnosis' into their search box.

Encouraging people to understand issues such as overdiagnosis is part of a movement to educate and empower citizens to become active partners in their care rather than passive patients. Many people in midlife are faced with difficult challenges in helping a parent with a number of conditions, and a much larger number of prescriptions, navigate through the maze of NHS services, often at a distance of 100 miles or more. We do not yet give people training or guidance on how to get the best from the NHS but there is a great book called *Staying Alive* by Phil Hammond, a GP and broadcaster, which has been written specifically to help you find solutions to common dilemmas such as how to find the right drug treatment for you and the right specialist and operation for you.

This approach is essential for decisions you face in midlife, whether or not to have an operation for back pain for example, but you also need to think ahead about decisions you might face at the end of life, or, even more worrying, decisions that might have to be made when you cannot express your preferences clearly. For this reason everyone aged 50 should start advance care planning.

Advance care planning

The dietary and lifestyle changes which have been discussed throughout this book are important for your health. However, they will also influence how your life ends and the way you die.

In addition to a will, you should make an 'advance care plan' setting out what you want to happen (and what you do not want to happen) should some serious, acute health problem, such as a major stroke, make it impossible to express yourself clearly.

Everyone who enters the second half of life should start advance care planning. The key principle is planning, not simply writing a plan – General Eisenhower said that 'plans are useless, but planning is indispensable' – but to keep thinking ahead and amending your plans as your condition or circumstances change.

The key step, and I cannot emphasise this enough, is at least to start the conversation. Of course, for many 50-year-olds this difficult conversation is not about their own future but about their parents and their end-of-life wishes or plans. The major review of end-of-life care conducted by the Royal College of Physicians and the Marie Curie charity which was published in 2015 found that in patients they studied, whose median age was 82, 'only 4% had documented evidence of an advance care plan made prior to admission to hospital'.

'What would Mum/Dad have wanted?' is often a mystery, particularly when summoned across the country to see a severely ill parent unable to communicate what they want and not having written anything down. Raising the need for advance care planning with an elderly parent is difficult, but that is not the focus of this book. Our focus is on people in midlife who should take steps to ensure that their children are not put in an awkward spot in 30 years' time.

Advance care planning covers three different aspects:

- What you want to happen – this is called an advance statement of wishes
- What you don't want to happen – this is called an advance decision to refuse treatment
- Who you want to have legal authority to act on your behalf if you lose the ability to make decisions for yourself – this is called a lasting power of attorney for health and welfare

There are good websites that guide you through this process, such as:

- www.compassionindying.org.uk
- www.mydirectives.com

This can be a delicate subject to discuss with your nearest and dearest but the more remote the possibility, the easier it is to raise. Start at 50, when the whistle blows for the second half of your life.

For many people in midlife life is tough, with financial and housing pressures creating a timescale that stretches only until next Friday. But think how you would like to see your-self in 10, 20 or 40 years' time. If you would like to be active and engaged with other people, helping friends and family, you need to start now, and one way to motivate yourself is to be clear about why you want to change.

Healthcare is what you do for yourself

The next most common type of healthcare is that which comes from friends and family and informal groups such as people who you get on with at work. Then from voluntary societies like Parkrun or Diabetes UK and commercial companies like Weight Watchers, Slimming World and Gymbox, and finally there are the public health and social services.

However, the basis of all successful change is how you feel, how much pressure you are under and how other organisations can help you improve your health, both short-term – next month, for example – and long-term, in 20 years' time.

In the 21st century clean, clear knowledge can transform the health of individuals and populations. At one time it seemed that the Internet would solve the problem because the Internet blew away the locked doors of medical libraries which patients were not allowed to enter. However, the Internet soon created another problem, replacing knowledge starvation with knowledge surfeit.

NHS Choices was designed to ensure that patients and citizens had access to the same knowledge as clinicians. Care is taken to use language that does not require clinical training to be understood, but this does not mean the information about risks and benefits is dumbed down. Your personal decision about whether or not to take a drug or to have a screening test or an operation does not require medical training. It requires you to understand:

- How the intervention will help you resolve your problem if it turns out well
- The probability of the intervention turning out well
- What happens if the intervention causes harm, which all tests and treatments can do, even in the best of hands
- The probability of the intervention causing harm

The NICE website also contains good information for patients and the public.

Another good source of advice is the series of Harvard Medical School Special Health Reports. You have to buy these but they go into detail about big issues such as suppleness or prostate cancer.

When a problem develops, raised blood pressure or type 2 diabetes for example, the websites of the relevant charity are reliable, clearly written and practical.

For many common conditions the Chartered Society of Physiotherapy website provides good, practical information at www.csp.org.uk.

National charities

There have been scandals in the papers about charity fundraising and this has given charities a bad image, but charities – big national charities and local charities – are great health services.

If you are told you have type 2 diabetes or high blood pressure you will find excellent information on the websites of Diabetes UK and the British Heart Foundation. If you are worried about cancer look at the Macmillan Cancer Support website, where you will also find very good information about the benefits of walking because they fund the Walking for Health programme in partnership with the Ramblers. If you have back or joint pain look at the Arthritis Research website and you will find practical, evidence-based advice as well as news of the latest research. For mental health, perhaps the problem for which the NHS is most variable, go to the websites for Mind and Rethink Mental Illness where there are support services as well as information.

Better health is too important to be left to the NHS alone. The NHS depends on charities, not to give money to the NHS, although the money they raise for research and development is very important, but to complement and supplement its services with the passion and care that charities bring.

4.

The Road Ahead: Reinvention and Revolution

Stop looking at midlife as the beginning of the end. Instead, start looking at midlife as the end of the beginning. Most people in midlife will reach 80 and many will live longer. Midlife is the kick-off to the second half of life – not full time.

Throughout this book, I have outlined the steps that you can take to feel better in the next few months. I have shown you the steps that will help you stay fitter and independent longer. The aim for most people is not to increase lifespan at any cost, but to increase the 'health span'. This is the quality of life. For many years, there was a concern that by introducing preventive medicine and extending lifespan, we were also increasing the period at the end of the life in which the individual was dependent on other people.

Reinvention

Midlife should not be seen as a time of inevitable decline. It can be a period in which you get fitter, lighter and younger. It is a period of your life in which you can improve your health and vitality, where you can find the energy to develop new knowledge and skills. It is also a time for planning your future, just like the time when you were leaving school – with all the excitement that comes with it.

In order to get there, however, you need to think about yourself. Here are some questions that may help you with this process:

Questions	Reflections
What am I really good at doing?	
Apart from the type of job I am doing at the moment, what other types of occupation are my strengths suited to?	
What skills would I like to develop?	
What subject or subjects would I like to know more about?	
If I could do something really different, what would that be?	
How has the experience of the last 20 years helped me deal more effectively with difficult situations?	
What would I like to be doing in 10 years' time?	
What do other people whose opinion I respect think I should do in a different direction?	

It is often helpful to discuss your reflections with someone else whose opinion you trust because you may have too rosy a view of your talents and potential (or, more likely, underestimate them). Some people have the resources to pay for a coach, or have a coach provided by their work, but you don't need to hire someone – just find a person you trust.

The second step is to set some objectives for yourself, not 'become a millionaire', but to think about how the world is changing and will change in the decade to come. Here are some questions that will help you identify key trends and reflect on their implications for you:

Key questions	Key trends	Implications for me
What will be the three most important global trends in the next decade?		
What will be the three most important trends affecting this country in the next decade?		
Which trends are most favourable to the industry I work in at present?		
Which trends threaten the industry I work in at present?		
What trends will play to my strengths and potential?		
What trends are likely to make my situation and prospects more difficult?		

Now you are in a position to relate your strengths and weaknesses to the changing world.

Obviously you need to have a plan for how you will improve your health – getting less stressed, sleeping better, getting fitter and eating healthier food. However, reinvention also involves changes in the way you live. Here is a list of routes you could follow:

- Change of job, but using the same set of skills
- Get a different type of job
- Develop a new set of skills through retraining or a degree
- Become self-employed
- Start a new business
- Become a volunteer

Midlife is an exciting time and a time when you're able to achieve all you've ever wanted. It's time to start your own personal revolution.

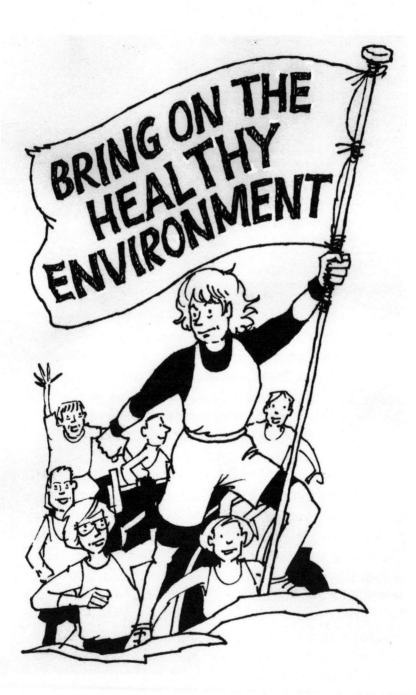

Join the revolution

A study in 2015 found that nearly half the days off sick from work were caused not by heart disease, type 2 diabetes or asthma but by stress, and of course people who are not in work suffer from the effects of stress too. But life doesn't have to be that way. A huge review of all the statistics about life expectancy in England, published in the famous medical journal the *Lancet* in 2015, reported that although life expectancy had increased in England by 6 years between 1990 and 2013, the difference in life expectancy between men in the wealthiest communities and men in the most deprived communities had not decreased in that time period. The difference between women in the two types of population had decreased from 7.2 years to 6.9 years, but the difference for men remained stubbornly at 8.2 years. Life doesn't have to be that way, so why is it that way?

The front page of the *Daily Mail* on 1 March 2016 carried the headline 'White Collar Pension Blow', the story being that 'white collar staff may be forced to wait longer for their pensions than manual workers' because of 'variations in life expectancy', but this difference is not related to the working conditions of the two groups.

In fact, if you want to stay healthy and live longer, an active job is a better option, as a famous study comparing the life expectancy of bus drivers and bus conductors showed, demonstrating that the conductors had lower risk of heart disease than the drivers. Neither is the difference solely the consequence of higher pay. Poverty is, of course, a cause of stress and depression but there are other more subtle causes of stress. A study of white-collar civil servants found that those who were higher up the ladder had a lower risk of heart attacks and the principal reason was not their higher pay but the fact that people lower down the ladder had less control over their working day.

In Part One there is information about steps you can take to reduce the causes of your stress and cope better with the reaction if you cannot deal with the source. That implies that stress is all due to you and to your inability to cope with your environment. Obviously there are factors in the physical environment that cause disease – air pollution, for example – but it is the social environment that is the cause of stress for most people: the environment at work, in their neighbourhood and in the family.

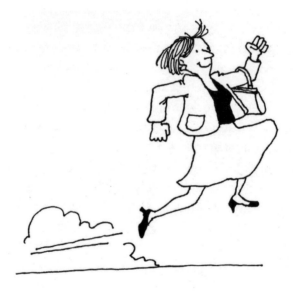

In March 2016 it was announced that the NHS, with the support of Public Health England, would build 76,000 'healthy homes' in ten towns; homes that were not only good for the family within them but also designed in a way that would encourage the development of a good physical and social environment. This is not an impossible dream. It is standard in some countries, notably Denmark. There is still the stress of work that has to be dealt with in a different way, principally by reducing bullying, which is unfortunately often seen by the bully as 'good management', but at least there is the realisation that a healthy environment can be created.

What is needed is:

- better affordable housing
- reduced fear of crime
- more green space
- lower priority for cars and higher priority for walking and cycling

This book has been written primarily to help you recognise that not everything that happens is due to ageing. It is to encourage you to take action to reduce your stress, improve your sleep, change your diet and start thinking about your fitness. However, you're also encouraged to change the world and take action to improve your lifestyle. Add health improvements to any club that you're a member of, and go and see your local councillor and MP to tell them what you think needs to be done. We need a social revolution to make sure that the health of the next generation is improved – and that needs to start now. It's time for the revolution.

Further Reading

Books about growing older and adapting well

The most important book is *The 100 Year Life* by Lynda Gratton and Andrew Scott, which sets out the challenge facing people in midlife, and those who are younger. An increasing proportion will reach 100, so a 35 or 40-year retirement is neither possible nor desirable. This book introduces the very clever concept of non-financial assets and the need to grow your assets through self-discovery, new challenges and training. *Call the Midlife* by Chris Evans is also good, particularly his call for people in midlife to talk about death and dying much more openly. His view on this subject is relevant for both sexes. For women in midlife, *The Longevity Book* by Cameron Diaz and Sandra Dark covers all aspects of ageing well, including the menopause. It is one of a number of books and articles which now emphasise that the aim for women of all ages is not skinniness but muscle.

Books on reducing stress

Manage Your Mind by Gillian Butler and Tony Hope and is an excellent guide to help you not only deal with stress and problems, but the subtitle is 'The Mental Fitness Guide', and it will also help you become more resilient. You might want to buy the key book on mindfulness – *Mindfulness*, by Mark Williams, Danny Penman and Jon Kabat-Zinn – as CD or on Kindle because you can then do the exercises to learn how to reduce stress and anxiety while listening to the audio version. It also has the excellent subtitle, 'A practical guide to finding peace in a frantic world'.

Books about keeping active and getting fitter

Try *Fast After 50* by Joe Friel for serious athleticism, of the triathlete variety. More realistic books for most people are *Younger Next Year* by Harry Lodge and *Older, Faster, Stronger* by Margaret Webb. For people who don't want, or have time, to get their kit off, try *Dr Gray's Walking Cure* by Muir Gray, and for people who are chained to their desk or computer screen, the following books give good advice to workers and their managers: *Is Your Chair Killing You?* by Kent Burden; *Sitting Kills, Moving Helps* by Joan Vernikos; *Get Up!: Why Your Chair Is Killing You and What You Can Do About It* by James Levine; *Deskbound: Standing Up to a Sitting World* by Kelly Starrett. These all contain good advice and suggestions for survival in a sitting world, for both workers and their managers.

Books about healthy eating

There are many books on diet – a bewildering number. Some like *Lean in 15* by Joe Wicks emphasise the importance of exercise as well as diet. Jamie Oliver's *Everyday Superfood* was written partly based on his reinvention of himself, with substantial weight loss at the age of 40. If you want to read about the benefits of a paleolithic diet, try *Fuel for Life* by Bear Grylls. For more conventional information, try *Sod It, Eat Well!* by Anita Bean and Muir Gray.

Books on making better medical decisions

Steve Woloshin, Lisa Schwartz and Gilbert Welch have written *Know Your Chances* – a clear and helpful book on how to understand and weigh up the options facing you. Gerd Gigerenzer's book, *Reckoning with Risk*, is also very clear and will help you think about your options when serious decisions have to be taken.

Acknowledgements

The Midlife Team is a small team of young doctors – Harpreet Sood, Nikki Kakani and Ben Maruthappu – who are not only very knowledgeable about the clinical and public health perspectives on midlife, but also fully understand how our message can flow into the digital media that Midlifers rely on.

Huw Armstrong and the Penguin Random House team have not only kept the project on track but also made intelligent contributions to the content and logic of the text.

Jackie Rosenthal and Jon Conibear of Offox Press have provided wisdom on the strategic direction of the book.

David Mostyn has shown his customary brilliance as an illustrator, capturing both the meaning and the spirit of the text.

Index

Index